"As a mother of three, I think this book should be in the home of all parents of older teens and young adults in today's world. It defines the stages of independence that should be taking place as our children grow up mentally and emotionally. It also clarifies the difference between being 'lazy' and not being ready—and helps young adults (and their parents!) build the future they want."
—Andrea M.

"A superb resource for parents who want to help young adult children develop the executive skills they need to reach their educational and career potential. No other book provides such a clear explanation of 'failure to launch' and converts scientific knowledge into practical problem-solving ideas. I can't praise this book enough—it's truly a gold mine of knowledge and tools for families."
—Mary V. Solanto, PhD, Department of Pediatrics, Zucker School of Medicine at Hofstra/Northwell

"This book will help you and your young adult get to know yourselves (and each other) better—and develop a plan to get 'unstuck.' Using your strengths and past successes, you can set goals and get the support you need to achieve them. I highly recommend this book for any parents and grown kids who need some practical help getting where they want to go!"
—Patricia O. Quinn, MD, coauthor of *Ready for Take-Off* and *On Your Own*

"The *Smart but Scattered* books are among the most useful and informative resources for managing executive skills problems. This one is chock-full of sound advice for young adults—including those who have ADHD—and their parents."
—Russell A. Barkley, PhD, ABPP, ABCN, author of *Taking Charge of ADHD*

Smart but Scattered—and Stalled

SMART but SCATTERED

—and Stalled

10 STEPS TO HELP YOUNG ADULTS
USE THEIR EXECUTIVE SKILLS
TO SET GOALS, MAKE A PLAN,
AND SUCCESSFULLY LEAVE THE NEST

Richard Guare, PhD

Colin Guare, MS

Peg Dawson, EdD

THE GUILFORD PRESS
NEW YORK   LONDON

For Megan, Colin, and Shannon
—DICK

For Jack, the Grammies, and Kate
—COLIN

For Steve, Aaron, and Isaac
—PEG

Copyright © 2019 The Guilford Press
A Division of Guilford Publications, Inc.
370 Seventh Avenue, Suite 1200, New York, NY 10001
www.guilford.com

Printed in the United States of America

This book is printed on acid-free paper.

Last digit is print number: 9   8   7   6   5   4   3   2   1

Library of Congress Cataloging-in-Publication Data is available from the publisher.

ISBN 978-1-4625-1554-7 (paperback) — ISBN 978-1-4625-3723-5 (hardcover)

Contents

Prologue   1
How I Got Stalled

Introduction   5
The Stepping Stones to Independence

STEP 1   Assess the Young Adult's Skills for Independence   15
The Executive in the Brain

STEP 2   Build a Foundation for Moving Forward   37
Motivation, Readiness, Respect, and Support

STEP 3   Identify a Realistic Direction   66
The Young Adult's Interests and Aptitudes

STEP 4   Plan How to Help—and Where Not To   89
Parents' Executive Skills and Respect for Boundaries

STEP 5   Set a Goal   120
Pull Everything Together and Evaluate Goodness of Fit

STEP 6   Make It Official   152
Use SMART Goals to Plan the Steps and Evaluate Progress

STEP 7   Make It Easier   177
Anticipate Problems and Intervene to Get Things Done

STEP 8 Get Creative to Tackle Specific Weaknesses   197

STEP 9 Seek Extra Help If You're Still Stalled   222

STEP 10 Learn from Your Success   239

Epilogue   251

APPENDIX Getting Help with Independent Living   253

Resources   264

Index   277

About the Authors   288

Prologue
How I Got Stalled

One day, in the first grade, I forgot to push in my chair . . .

Right now, I am sitting in the forward sleeping area of the *Ellen Diane*, a 45-foot fishing boat that I have been a deckhand on for 7 months. It is a dragger, meaning that we drag a net attached to the boat by long cables to catch cod, dogfish, flounder, lobsters, and, if we are lucky, a few scallops, which I shuck and eat raw right on the boat.

But there is also ample downtime for even a hall-of-fame procrastinator like me to feel guilty for not attempting to describe what led me here, at least the parts that inform the topic of this book. Not that I haven't tried, of course; as I said, for 7 months I've been riding around the waters constituting the local fishing grounds south of the Isles of Shoals, off the coast of New Hampshire. I read books on seamanship and solo circumnavigations of the world by men in small sailboats. I borrowed (stole) an old Audubon field guide from my parents' house; I study it and take woefully inadequate pictures with my iPhone for later reference. I still can't distinguish between the common tern and the roseate tern.

I read stories by Joyce Carol Oates and John Cheever (my favorite). I quit smoking. I listen to recordings of Yale lectures on psychology, I listen to Lady Gaga. On five separate occasions I read the first 10 pages of Joyce's *Ulysses* and fall asleep. I text my girlfriend and play Scramble with Friends with strangers. I talk to the captain or the scientists that sometimes ride with us to do research. I break an 8-day streak of unassisted completions of the *Boston Globe* crossword because I don't know what oleo is. I start smoking again. I whale-watch. I make plans to buy a sextant and teach myself celestial navigation. I seriously contemplate taking up whittling, but don't because it would be too much of a cliché (and not because I lack artistic talent in the way that an amoeba lacks a spinal cord). I even do a little writing.

But I don't start this working on this book. I don't really think about it; I might even try not to. Never mind that I have already written one, so I know it is possible. Or that Chris and Kitty, our editors, are thoughtful and encouraging and relentlessly optimistic and reassuring about our projects. Or that as we approach our first deadline, the communicative equivalent of the theme to *Jaws* (which I've watched eight times in the last 2 months), will become the undercurrent of almost every interaction with my father/coauthor. Or that I want to be a writer, in some sense of the word, and that this is an unbelievable opportunity that I should cherish and be rigorously devoted to. I am not ungrateful for it; in fact, it's proof positive that despite myself, the love, support, gentle nudges, and hard kicks in the ass from my friends and family have landed me right-side-up and none the worse for wear after 25 years. I am not afraid to admit it.

So why haven't I started until now? When I look at that question, it occurs to me that this isn't the first, or second, or hundredth, or thousandth time I've asked it. I suppose the reason, in part, is the bane of everyone from eighth graders to Nobel laureates: writer's block. The job description of a writer has within itself all the ingredients necessary to cook up problems: long spans of unsupervised time punctuated by a few incredibly important landmarks. No memos, no CEOs or middle management, no time clock with the exception of an occasional note from an editor.

At this point you might have a few questions, like "Colin, how does writer's block connect with the themes of this book? My child isn't a writer, so how does this information apply?" Well, it applies because for me the issue goes well beyond writer's block. Writing happens to be one of those tasks (but not the only one by a long shot) that requires sustained attention, the ability to resist distraction; task initiation rather than procrastination; time management and a sense of time urgency; planning; and organization. In short, writing puts a high premium on what we call the mind's "executive skills." So while writer's block is real, for me it's also a circumstantial term for the more generic issue of weak executive skills. And as you'll see, the effects extend far beyond my current bout of "writer's block." For me, writing is only the most recent (and most demanding) vehicle to highlight these skills.

When I was 6, in Mrs. Davis's first-grade class, I once forgot to push my chair in after getting up from my desk. I don't remember the date or what I was wearing, the sky didn't fall that day, and I wasn't expelled, and Mrs. Davis didn't drum my knuckles with a ruler (she was a kind and firm teacher, and scary enough without the threat of corporal punishment). The chair was eventually pushed in, and the moment passed unnoticed. I mention it as a playful anecdote that I daydream about; if I could time-travel, or call through time and leave an answering machine message ("voicemail" wasn't commonly used in 1993, remember?) telling my parents to make absolutely sure I always pushed my chair in—if that happened, I imagine that all my subsequent issues would never have materialized, not drastically changing my life but just giving myself a bit of a tune-up. Because the next day it happened again. It happened again, and again, and again, to the point that it became part of an informal report card that Mrs. Davis gave to my parents every week, and by the end of the year chair-pushing-in wasn't the only thing being graded. "Talking out" (offering unsolicited comments) was added to the list. Elementary school was an era of field testing by myself, my teachers, and my mom and dad. Problems would crop up—leaving things behind, interrupting people, not "using my time wisely"—and we would collectively develop strategies to fix them. Even though academics was never a problem, an awful lot of the rest of my life was. And now here I sit, 25 years old, without a personal rudder or charted course into adult life.

Over the next decade-plus, in elementary school and through my sophomore year in high school, I brought home good report cards. But my affinity for reading on my own and independent learning was a mixed blessing that mostly masked my deficiencies in the executive skills necessary for managing life: organization, planning, time management, initiating and following through on tasks and goals, and more. These deficiencies became increasingly evident. Once I had my driver's license I was late all the time; late to school, for dinner with my family or a date, sports, friends. My failure to complete homework and commit to the time needed for junior year's more specific, rigorously taught subjects led to a drop in some of my grades, despite good scores on AP tests. When physics entered my curriculum, I took a nosedive, doing all right at first but quickly mistaking the ease of that initial survey material for what the rest of the course would be like. I ended up with a D, but because the rest of my grades provided a lot of padding for my GPA, I subscribed to a type of mental math that allowed me to shrug it off and that served me just as badly once I got to college.

Besides failing to grasp that the academic landscape in all college courses would resemble that AP physics course, I took advantage of the lack of structure plus a lack of self-regulation to overindulge in alcohol and other extracurricular activities at the expense of everything else. By the end of the first semester I left with a GPA so low I thought it was mathematically impossible.

It didn't end there either; I spent the next few years at a different school, doing marginally better or worse, taking full or partial class loads as I wanted or was allowed. I was like an actor with a breakout movie who mistook raw talent (my high school performance) for commitment and effort. My next big movie was a flop. Then I underperformed in a couple of B movies and did a celebrity reality show before taking a needed hiatus.

For me, that was leaving school altogether and working full time. I moved away to Nantucket, an island that is a popular summertime destination, and worked landscaping for almost 2 years. My job confronted me with things that I could wrap my head around and learn——how to pay bills, do taxes without my parents' help, go grocery shopping, split chores among roommates, save money—many of the things I think make people "feel" adult. I ultimately felt this phase of my life had run its course and moved back home, where I floundered for another year trying to find a job and a sense of purpose. Finally, I ended up on this boat. It's not where I saw myself staying, and it wasn't what my parents had envisioned for me when they dropped me off at that 4-year college a few years earlier. I had learned some of the skills of self-sufficiency, but independent adult life was still a work in progress. What helped me gradually find some traction were the concrete steps of goal setting and achievement, the collaborative support, and the skill-building ideas you'll find in this book. Oh, and pretty great parents.

COLIN GUARE, 2014

Introduction
The Stepping Stones to Independence

This book is not a story about my son, Colin. It's a story about people like Colin, young adults who are smart but scattered, who struggle to find a direction or a destination—or, if they have a destination, can't seem to get there. It's about how to get past the "failure to launch"—a growing trend among young adults to either stay or move back home with their parents. It's about dealing with the financial and emotional costs, the frequent conflicts, and the resulting low self-esteem, anxiety, and depression that plague young adults who are stalled in their progress toward independence and the parents who are trying to help them leave the nest.

Do you have a son or daughter who has bounced back from college (perhaps more than once, like Colin) and is spending a lot more than the anticipated few months at a going-nowhere minimum-wage job while trying to figure out what to do next? Does your 22-year-old son still have trouble doing his own laundry, getting up in time for work, and avoiding checking account overdrafts—despite the fact that he's living with you rent-free? Are you watching with growing distress and helplessness as your energetic, creative daughter realizes her BA hasn't prepared her for a career that interests her at all, but she has no idea what the best direction is for her and she seems to be reacting by hiding under the covers?

Throughout this book, you will read the stories of a number of young adults in addition to Colin's. These individuals are composites of the many young men and women we have worked with, and you will likely identify with various aspects of their circumstances as they move toward independence. Set off from the rest of the text, you'll find Colin's first-person account of his own journey.

Smart but stalled young adults often experience academic failure. They might appear unmotivated, lacking a sense of purpose or a "passion." They sometimes seem satisfied with the immediate gratifications that they can extract from web surfing, video games, online social media, television, or, more troubling, drugs and alcohol. They are either living at home or dependent on parents for more of their living expenses and for a longer time than you or they ever envisioned. As the *Wall Street Journal* reported at the end of 2016, 40% of young Americans were living with parents or other relatives in 2015—a 75-year-high. There are myriad economic and social reasons for this trend, and it's beyond the scope of this book to analyze them all. Our goal is to help you figure out what's going on in your young adult's mind, in your own mind, and in the relationship between you that's keeping your adult child stalled. Failures to launch are usually complex problems that may involve deficiencies in the mind's executive skills (your child's and your own), along with attitudes, expectations, and dynamics in the family that have developed over the adult child's life.

If you read our books about younger people—*Smart but Scattered* and *Smart but Scattered Teens*—you know that executive skills are part of the brain development that takes place over the first 25 or 30 years of life and that some kids experience weaknesses or delays in developing some or all of these skills. (In fact, we're all weaker in some skills than in others, and therefore everyone could be seen as having executive skills deficits to some degree.) As a result, they need extra help with being organized, on time, focused, and in control. As they mature, life's demands on these skills increase, and even if you've been substituting for your son or daughter's frontal lobes so far—or using our ideas to help your child strengthen weaker skills—continuing to do so not only becomes less and less practical but is also counterproductive when the goal is to nudge your child toward independence.

By the time they are 18 or 21 or 25, the world they live in expects young adults to start doing things for themselves. But young adults with executive skill deficiencies often get lost in wanderings, disappointments, and "failures" as life tasks get more complicated and require more attention and planning. As Colin articulates so clearly and candidly in this book, he has experienced significant executive skill challenges throughout his life, beginning in early childhood. The data? Forgotten rules in first grade; my regular visits to lost-and-found; unmet academic expectations; detentions and suspensions; college dropout × 3; unpaid bills, rent, and taxes; alcohol, DWI; low self-esteem, anxiety, depression.

You may no longer be making regular visits to the school lost-and-found for your child or spending your evenings at your child's elbow to be sure she completes homework, yet you're still picking up after your adult child, paying his or her bills, and issuing reminders about tasks to be done. Or the young adult is taking care of chores and paying bills, but seems to be perfectly happy to enhance his lifestyle by living at home, and you're wondering if he's going to be there until you're 80. At this point you've probably come up with dozens of career suggestions (too many?), offered bounteous support (too much?), and alternated between patient understanding (too patient?) and tough love (too tough?). Your adult child probably isn't happy about the current situation either, and your relationship might be described as an uneasy peace too often broken by blowups or tense standoffs.

How Do You Get Out of This Trap?

You need specific steps that you can take together, one at a time, to set a realistic goal and work toward achieving it. This is what we offer in this book. When adult children get stalled on their way to independence, there's a very good chance that they haven't started with a goal that (1) is realistically achievable, (2) parent and adult child can agree on, and (3) is the *young adult's* choice. But a history of false starts, missteps, disappointments, and resentments can rob both the young adult and the parents of any confidence that they know how to choose an appropriate goal and how to achieve it. In this book you'll have the opportunity to step back, away from the conflict and confusion, and use proven, practical tools to identify a goal and make progress toward it in a way that leads to a measure of independence that you can build on over time. And this process, we've found, is helpful to all stalled young adults—even those with relatively minor executive skill issues—and their parents. Stalls can be caused by a confluence of factors that need to be taken into account (see the box below).

WHAT CAUSES YOUNG ADULTS TO STALL ON THEIR WAY TO INDEPENDENCE?

Your car can stall for a variety of reasons. So can your young adult:

- Executive skills weaknesses
- Unrealistic expectations
- Undefined goals
- Goals dictated by parents

- Lack of confidence or fear of failure
- Too much parental help and too many rescues
- Too little parental help and a rigid "sink-or-swim" approach by parents
- Too much comfort right where they are
- No experience with handling the practical tasks of independent living
- Depression, anxiety, or other mental health challenges

We put executive skills challenges at the top of the list because it's tough to achieve independence when executive skills aren't fully developed, but any or all of the other factors can halt forward movement for any young adult. We address all of these factors throughout the program.

What to Expect from This Program

We—Peg and Dick—have worked with smart but scattered kids for much of our professional lives, most recently developing a successful model for coaching students with executive skills deficits. Based on that work, our work with parents and their smart but scattered children, and Colin's experience, we have come up with 10 steps that parents and stalled young adults can follow to start the young adult on the path to independence. Here's how it works:

Step 1: Figure out whether the young adult has the fundamental, brain-based skills for independence. Odds are the young adult has some executive skills challenges that are at the root of being stuck. Identify these and you immediately call off the "blame game" and can start figuring out how to work with the adult child's strengths and weaknesses to get out of the quagmire.

Step 2: Find out whether you're both ready to move forward. You'd probably both reflexively say "Of course I am!," but not all parents are as ready to let go as they think they are, and not all young adults are motivated to take on adult responsibilities along with the accompanying adult freedoms. Figure out how you both define "independence" and what you want. Assess how ready and willing you are. Bump up motivation and readiness for change, polish your mutual respect, and commit to collaborating. That's the foundation for launching.

Step 3: Identify the young adult's aptitudes and preferences. We've seen kids make education and career choices based on their friends' interests, their parents' expectations, or the latest trends—with no consideration of what *they* want. We've coached young adults who aspire to careers that require talents they don't have or skills and knowledge they're not motivated to acquire. Here's a chance to find out what a particular young adult really prefers, whether she has what she needs to go for it, and, if not, whether she's willing and able to spend the time and effort to become prepared.

Step 4: Identify what the parent can bring to the table. Find out what your own executive skills look like and you'll not only get an idea of where conflicts might arise between you and your adult child but also how you can complement each other in the goal-setting and goal-reaching processes. Here's where you also use tools to dig deeper into where and how you as parent can provide support and where and how you should step back.

Step 5: Set a goal. Here you'll find tools to pull together all the information you've gathered so far to set a good goal. Illustrations will show that a goal that creates any measurable change toward independence is a good one— something as modest as pitching in on chores and taking responsibility for self-care to more ambitious targets, like working toward long-term career goals. It all depends on where the young adult is starting out.

Step 6: Break it down to make it happen. A goal is only as good as the steps you take to reach it. Here are the tools and strategies for breaking a goal into manageable objectives, tracking progress, and reviewing the overall direction you're taking.

Step 7: Anticipate trouble and do some advance work to overcome challenges. Executive skill weaknesses cause predictable problems. You can head them off by modifying the environment in which tasks will be done to reach the goal—by altering the task, by altering the surroundings, or by planning to get help from others. There are also ways to build the weakest executive skills to bolster the chances of success.

Step 8: Get creative to disarm specific skill weaknesses. Here Colin describes the typical derailments that can occur for those with specific executive skills weaknesses. Weak in response inhibition? Don't go to your favorite bar to watch the game with most of your paycheck in your pocket. Trouble with time management? Use any of the widely available tech tools to help you stay on schedule. We offer a wealth of suggestions born of experience.

Step 9: Get extra help if you need it. Sometimes goal achievement is thwarted despite your best efforts. Your best bet if that happens is to review carefully whether any progress has been made and whether the time frame is what you both planned for. If not, can you tweak the plan? How much time and effort you want to put into trying alternatives depends on your tolerance for continuing to be stuck. If you feel like you're ending up back where you started, try consulting a coach. If the young adult seems plagued by depression or anxiety, get a mental health evaluation and whatever help is needed.

Step 10: Learn from success. Be sure to mark and capitalize on whatever has been working. You'll read here about what worked for young adults we've described throughout the book and may want to consider adopting some of their tactics as well. And, of course, there's room for learning from your mistakes (and those of others) too.

Tips for Using This Book

Work together. This book is for both of you. Read it separately if you wish, but work through the steps together. It's a collaborative journey. A stalled young adult will need help from a parent (or other adult who knows the young adult well), and a parent should never attempt to make the decisions laid out in the 10 steps for the adult child—that would run completely counter to the idea of passing the baton and promoting independence.

Work through the steps in order. The program provides a foundation of knowledge that you need to set a goal and then actions to take that will keep you on track for meeting the goal. Don't try to set a goal without the foundational information gathering or to use the strategies in the later steps without having a goal and a plan for reaching it. Steps 7 and 8 are a little more flexible, offering a toolkit of methods that you can apply while working toward the goal, not necessarily in a rigid order. Step 9 is there for you if you get stalled again but might not be needed, and Step 10 is a wrap-up for marking success and using what works throughout life—when you've achieved the goal or are well on your way, you deserve to celebrate newfound independence.

Keep your minds open. You're likely to learn a lot about yourselves and each other while you follow these steps toward independence (independence for both of you!). Realizing how each of you may have contributed to the stalling of the adult child's self-sufficiency may cause occasional discomfort. You very well might have to alter your expectations, recognize pipe dreams for what they are, and revel in the success of finding a path to what the young adult really wants out of life.

Even though my wife and I had set up a variety of systems to help Colin manage school, we somehow didn't anticipate his transition to college being a problem. Why? I think fundamentally because I wanted to believe the dream that I had, that a lot of us have—you know, your kid goes off to college, succeeds, finds a career, and lives independently and happily. Did Colin have that dream? In retrospect, apparently not.

> I didn't have a dream. I had ideas, vague thoughts, stuff that was transient. I had interests that were diverse, but nothing that felt sustainable. I don't think any of that was abnormal for a teenager. I cared a lot about what people would think and assumed that what people wanted was a plan, a respectable and aspirational plan. So I developed one and it went sideways, failed terribly, and I didn't know what to do after that. Caring about what other people think wasn't the problem; everyone does that. Assuming I knew what they thought or what their values were was the problem, I really believed I could predict how my choices would be judged. At that age, and when I didn't or couldn't stop to think hard about who "they" even are, using that system to make decisions was an especially flawed version of putting the cart before the horse.

I guess when you plant an idea from early on and talk about it, nurture it, you hope it becomes the child's dream. And maybe he believes or pretends it's his dream because he doesn't want to disappoint you. A lot of things conspire to reinforce the dream—the child's teachers, his friends' parents, his high school friends, and the working- and middle-class notions about what is necessary for success. In any case, it was easy for me as his dad to sign on to because I was the first person in my family to graduate from college and I believed my parents when they said it was important. And that's what we told Colin, that's what he heard in his schools and community, and that's what his friends were doing, and he was smart. So I pretty much whistled past the potential problems, and we took him off to the college and the major he had chosen and hoped for the best.

When Colin dropped out and decided to move to the island and work in landscaping, it wasn't what we had pictured. But he felt his nearly 2 years on the island was transformative, as it was for my wife and me. He had managed completely on his own, and we realized, and, perhaps more important, accepted that he could make a life for himself; it seemed he was pretty happy with doing something that was unrelated to what we had thought was the goal that we had all signed on for—finish school in 4 years, get a job, and get on the path to some career. So for us, the new reality was that whatever he wanted to do, as long as he was reasonably happy with it and able to manage his life, was okay for us.

There were stops and starts after that, and Colin and I will tell you about them where they're relevant in the steps laid out in the rest of this book and in the Epilogue. Suffice it to say for now that Colin has weathered it all. And he's emerged (from his father's unbiased perspective) as a remarkable young adult. The data? He is an accomplished creative writer; he has an ethic and talent for work that spans an unusual range—roofer, landscaper, trawler deckhand, behavior specialist for children with severe autism; and he had the 10-plus-year perseverance to continue working toward a college degree. And he's one of the kindest, most intelligent, and open-minded people I know.

It's our wish—mine, Colin's, and Peg's—that your journey is ultimately as satisfying.

Before You Start . . .

Taking the 10 steps that follow represents a shift for parent and adult child in how each of you thinks and behaves regarding roles and expectations. Before you start, think about the following questions.

Parents:

✓ How are you currently defining "independence," and is your definition realistic?

✓ Are you helping your adult child move forward or unwittingly making staying put too attractive or easy?

✓ Have you thought about what kind of help you're willing and able to provide, under what conditions, to help your child make progress?

✓ Do you think you have the executive skills yourself to help rather than hinder?

Young Adults:

✓ Are you motivated and ready to become more independent?

✓ Do you know what you really want to do—what type of work, what type of living arrangement, what geographical location you prefer?

✓ Do you have the talents and skills to pursue what you want?

✓ Are you willing and able to build the skills and knowledge to get where you want to go?

Both:

✓ Can you let go of prior expectations and assumptions and start your journey with an open mind?

✓ Can you come to agreement on a goal even if it's not the ideal you were envisioning?

✓ Can you set a realistic goal and a realistic time frame for achieving it?

STEP 1

Assess the Young Adult's Skills
for Independence
The Executive in the Brain

Terry has an appointment for a job interview and, as is typical for her, she gets a late start. On the drive she tries to make up lost time and is stopped for speeding. Terry resists the urge to argue with the police officer and instead apologizes for her mistake and briefly explains why it happened. She gets off with a warning.

Jackson, who is struggling with completing his degree, has a short paper due for an online course he is taking. He starts to research topics on his computer but takes a break to check how his fantasy football team is doing, and 2 hours later he still doesn't have a topic.

Tirone started a new job a week ago. He's supposed to punch in by 7:00 A.M. He's ready on time but as usual can't find his wallet or car keys. He arrives late and gets a written warning from his boss.

All of these young adults are stalled, in one fashion or another, as a result of significant weaknesses in one or more executive skills. Terry evidences both weak and strong executive skills. It looks like she doesn't have a good sense of time, but she is good at controlling her feelings. Jackson seems to have issues with getting started and maintaining his focus. And Tirone apparently struggles with making plans and keeping belongings in order.

Introducing Executive Skills

So what exactly do we mean by "executive skills," and why do they have so much power over us? The executive skills in the brain help us reach our goals, whether they're as simple and short term as getting to an appointment on time or as complex and long term as getting a college degree. In fact, we need these executive skills to choose our goals to begin with. Then we need them to regulate or guide our behavior in a way that makes it likely that we will reach those goals. On the flip side, they are the skills that help us avoid the behaviors that will derail our progress.

When some people hear the term "executive skills," they think it refers to skills needed by a successful business executive. There is some overlap: planning, task initiation, and focus are used by both the business executive and the young adult (and the rest of us) to accomplish goals. But the term in fact comes from the neuroscience literature and refers to a set of brain-based skills that are required for humans to *execute*, or successfully perform, tasks. When a young adult is stuck, in spite of having academic and work skills as well as preferences that suggest reasonable fit with a goal, it is likely that weaknesses in executive skills play a significant role because these skills are essential for successful goal accomplishment *and* independent living.

Executive skills are the brain-based skills needed to perform tasks.

If your son or daughter has a passion for (or even a sustained interest in) a particular subject, craft, vocation, or career path, you might wonder why the young adult is stalled. How can a person who's been a valued pet sitter and tireless volunteer at the local pet shelter, and really seems to be a dog or cat whisperer, never seem to get even close to the avowed dream of becoming a veterinarian? Why would the kid who's been talking about being a master game developer since the age of 9 not work hard to learn how to code? Sometimes knowing what you like to do and want to pursue isn't enough. It's also not always enough to have the talent or aptitude a goal requires. If interest and aptitude were sufficient for goal attainment, many more young adults would be in their dream jobs or would have finished college. Colin, for example (National Honor Society, SAT scores from the 96th to the 99th percentile), would have finished college and likely been involved in writing about language, literature, or politics. Clearly, he, as do many young adults, had the interests and aptitude to reach those goals.

But goal attainment requires additional skills. In pursuit of a goal we need to be able to develop a plan, the road map, for how to travel toward the goal.

And we need to be able to sustain the attention necessary to maintain focus on the road. We need to have the flexibility and emotional control to manage any roadblocks that get in the way, as well as the time management skills to balance the other day-to-day responsibilities that come along. Collectively these are what we call the brain's "executive skills."

Executive Skills Weaknesses in Action

Many stuck young adults exhibit problems like Terry's, Jackson's, or Tirone's over and over, so that they never seem to get where they want to go. But as a parent who wants to see your child succeed, it can be hard to attribute the failure to launch to brain-based problems rather than concluding that your child isn't trying hard enough, doesn't care enough, or is just naturally lazy. This chapter will give you and your young adult a chance to see where your son or daughter's executive skills stand so you have an inkling of how any weaknesses are keeping the young adult stuck.

You may have been dealing with your child's executive skills deficits for as long as you can remember. Terry had more "tardies" on her report cards than any of her elementary school classmates, and she typically had to pull an all-nighter to hastily slap together papers due in high school. Jackson is his family's "airhead," always needing to have instructions repeated, constantly wandering away from half-finished chores and projects—even the ones he was supposedly interested in. And Tirone was often compared to the Charles Schultz Pig-Pen character, with a cloud of dust, flotsam, and jetsam trailing him everywhere he went. He never put anything back where it belonged, so his environment was a chronic mess. But for the most part these three got by. Terry did get to school and get her papers in, with a little help from her parents. Jackson's pediatrician said he might have a mild case of attention-deficit/hyperactivity disorder (ADHD) and suggested some tools like electronic reminders to keep him moving forward on assignments and other tasks. His parents often served as his frontal lobes, and with help from them and his teachers, he graduated from high school with a 3.0 grade point average (GPA). Tirone has cost his family a lot of money for cell phones, new sets of keys, and sports equipment to replace what he's lost. They've started keeping a tally of these expenses, and he's supposed to be reimbursing them a little at a time out of his paycheck. They had hoped that feeling obligated to them would make him more conscientious about this latest in a string of jobs, but now they wonder if he just doesn't care about his family.

Colin "got by" too:

In the early years (from elementary school through sophomore year of high school) my natural abilities had the side effect of hiding my executive skills deficiencies; I could effectively close the gap of poor life management by just being smart. This had the twofold effect of not only leading others to believe I possessed these skills when I didn't, but also allowing me to make it successfully through school without ever having to work on them. Yes, the chair pushing in and talking out were examples of issues identified by my teachers and parents, but it's difficult for adults to assess whether these are temporary, isolated issues ("kids being kids," or "boy brains" as my mother calls it) or whether they foreshadow more serious issues down the road. Some present-day school systems, both public and private, have begun to implement curricula that help develop these skills by teaching them and monitoring student performance. In my case, some solutions worked better than others, some problems were more persistent than others. Some I've simply grown out of (biting my nails); others are works-in-progress (to-do lists and other reminders). Sometimes issues arose completely out of the blue, but in many cases my executive skills problems correlated to universal teenage milestones. Even if I had a time machine, I doubt I could have been punctual for anything between 2003 and 2005, for example.

Junior year of high school was when I began to struggle significantly. Similar to college, junior year at my high school marks an informal end to a general, student-body-wide course load and begins asking students to commit to more specific, rigorously taught subjects. It required a realignment of my learning style; no longer is a good handle on general topics adequate for good grades; now time and energy must be devoted to lengthy studies of very particular disciplines.

Spoiler alert: I didn't realign. Between junior and senior year I took four advanced placement (AP) classes: U.S. history, U.S. government, physics 1, and English. I love(d) history, government, and English, and it showed; my AP test scores on those were 4, 4, and 5, respectively (where 1 is the lowest score and 5 is the highest score). What's more interesting, though, is that my grades in those classes didn't reflect this result at all. I didn't fail, but in comparison to my classmates I was middle-of-the-road at best. The results were a catch-22 of my own design, because it somewhat validated my views at the time that if the purpose of the course was to do well on the test, then why do my missed homework assignments matter? I got A's and B's on the tests, so give me A's and B's for the class because I clearly did what was asked of me.

The real warning sign that I would struggle in college was my physics class. The first month or so was a breeze, designed to refresh us and lay down fundamental concepts that would be important later. I took this month as an indicator of the class as a whole, and proceeded to ignore most of the material, learning only enough to complete daily and weekly assignments. I had no real interest in physics, I was a casually proficient math student at best, the course was there, so I took it to boost my college résumé. By Christmas break I had floundered completely. The course accelerated quickly, and for the first time I was confronted by something that I didn't like, didn't understand, and couldn't master or even comprehend without diligent study.

My response? In short, I simply bailed out. I ignored the class as much as I could. I had done some of this in the past, but this was senior year AP physics; my teacher was wonderful, but he wasn't there to babysit me or liaison with my parents. By the time things came to a head and my guidance counselor notified them that I was in serious trouble, it was too late in my mind. I suppose I could have gritted my teeth and tried to make up all the work, but it seemed insurmountable.

Later it became obvious how shortsighted it was for me to dismiss the impact of homework on my performance, and clearly I completely missed the boat on the secondary lessons and skills that homework is trying to reinforce: consistent, independent completion of work on time. At the time it was annoying, but the end result was positive, so I ignored it; in retrospect it was a perfect dichotomy for understanding how and why I would struggle down the road.

My wife and I* were certainly aware of Colin's issues with executive skills, and from elementary school through high school we put various monitoring systems in place that provided us with timely information about academics and behavior in school and we set up a variety of systems to help him manage school. These included limits on access to distractions (TV, Internet, phone,

---

*Whenever we use the authorial "I," outside the vignettes about Colin and others, Richard Guare is speaking.

etc.) and making access to things he wanted (TV, Internet, free time, use of the car) contingent on acceptable school performance and behavior. From middle school through the end of high school he and I had more than our share of confrontations and conflicts about what he saw as unnecessary intrusions into his life. But he got through high school relatively unscathed, so from my perspective the system worked. At least until he went off to college, as Colin recalls:

In high school, my parents made access to gratification somewhat dependent on the effort I put into my studies. No effort = no results = no privileges (roughly). But when I got to college, the timely monitoring and red-flag systems that my parents and teachers had had in place were now absent. Hence, I could tell myself (and I did) that I could catch up or recover anytime with a little effort. The second element, time distortion, contributed to this illusion so that I underestimated the amount of time that I needed to put into coursework. My courses seemed easy at first, making it easier for me to skip just that one class or teacher assistant (TA) session. And I overestimated the amount of time that I had available since the whole semester was in front of me.

Tempus edax rerum—time, in fact, gradually devoured my opportunities. Once I fell behind, the amount of effort that I perceived necessary to catch up was daunting, So I defaulted to immediate gratification to escape the uncomfortable thoughts and comfort myself with the continuing belief that I still had time. The system works until the piper calls. After that point I saw a mountain of coursework that I'd never come back from, and ignored it because of the perceived effort, stress, and shame that it gave me.

In reality, at that point, I could have acted—met with my professors and counselors, mitigated the damage. And it probably would have worked; most college educators do have a sympathetic ear for students who temporarily forget what their job is, and are willing to cut them some slack. But I was the person who ran up his credit card to the limit of instant gratification, and instead of proactively contacting a debt consultant, I sat in my room biting my fingernails until the collection agency came knocking. The immediate context provided a ready-made distraction and escape. Things we don't want to do are always perceived as more difficult than they actually are. As I put off catching up on my classwork and seeing professors during office hours to patch up my attendance record, the perceived effort I thought it would take increased exponentially. Thus, the point at which I simply conceded that the semester was a total loss was a lot earlier than it was in reality. And by the time I made this known to my parents, the semester really was in dire straits.

Ultimately, I probably put more effort into a failed attempt at resurrecting the semester than it would have taken to fix it when I first acknowledged it as a problem. This is a pattern of behavior that has been with me for much of my life, but again, it didn't necessarily reveal itself until the game changed and the stakes were much higher than before.

Are Executive Skills Deficits Stalling Your Young Adult?

For all of our sons and daughters, the reality is that looming adulthood changes the landscape. Obviously, leaving the nest for an independent life means being largely self-sufficient: No more parents coming to the rescue with trips to the lost-and-found. No more endless financial backup—they start to peter out. No more authorities cutting your son or daughter slack for repeated recklessness and carelessness because he or she is "just a kid." These supports are rarely withdrawn abruptly or all at once, but the young adult's goal is to gradually move toward doing without them. To ensure that progress can be made in that direction, you have to know where the young adult's executive skills strengths and weaknesses lie. Weaknesses can hold your child back. Strengths can help him or her move forward.

Your adult child could be stuck for a variety of reasons, and maybe executive skills weaknesses aren't significant. This book will help you look at the complex matrix of factors typically involved, including lack of motivation and readiness for independence, ambivalence from parents, feeling too comfortable where they are, not knowing what they like or are good at, and wanting something that seems hopelessly out of reach. But we strongly suggest that the young adult and his or her parents complete the Executive Skills Questionnaire on pages 31–33 anyway. Whether you've never heard of executive skills or you both believe you know which executive skills are a problem for your child, you'll find that the questionnaires help you set aside a lot of assumptions that may have been stifling your ability to look at the situation clearly and fairly and give you some ideas for moving forward.

For parents and young adults who are not familiar with executive skills, the following information will provide you with an understanding of what executive skills are, how they develop, and the key role they play in the young adult's journey to independence. (If you've read one of our books about executive skills, *Smart but Scattered, Smart but Scattered Teens,* or *The Smart but Scattered Guide to Success,* the information below may serve as a refresher, or if you're knowledgeable in this area, you may want to skip ahead to the questionnaires, where you can begin to apply this information to your young adult.)

How We Acquire Executive Skills

How do executive skills develop? There are two main contributors to the development of executive skills: neurobiology and experience. The neurobiological contribution begins with genetics. The genes you inherited from your parents affected your own executive skills development, and the genes you passed on to your young adult likewise have impacted his or her skills. And as with other skills, such as language development, the brain is hardwired at birth for executive skills to develop. At birth, these skills exist only as *potential*. Newborns don't speak, and they don't display executive skills. But as long as no pre- or early postnatal disease or trauma has occurred to damage this neurological equipment, these skills will develop.

Beyond that, the environment and the experiences in that environment play a major role in executive skills development. A biologically or physically toxic environment can alter the neurobiological substrate underlying executive skills. Environmental toxins include anything from lead exposure to poverty to child abuse. And there is growing evidence that significant psychosocial stress (conflict in the family, sustained negative interactions with the child) can also adversely impact the brain and hence executive skills development. But if we assume reasonably normal neurobiological equipment and the absence of negative genetic or environmental factors, then executive skills development proceeds more or less as it is supposed to, starting at a very early age.

> The experiences we have in our environment while growing up have a strong influence on how our executive skills develop.

The infant enters the world with a brain primed for interaction with people and the environment. And she learns from those interactions and adjusts her behavior as a result. When, at 8 months, the infant sees a cat disappear into another room and crawls after it, she is demonstrating rudimentary executive skills: visual working memory, initiation, attention, even goal-directed persistence. At this age, though, she doesn't have all the executive skills she needs to be safe. If she comes to an ungated set of stairs, she may start down them without any thought about the consequences. She lacks inhibition, so you as a parent intervene and lend yours to the situation. This is a very early example of a process that will go on between you and your child for a long time—25 or more years in fact, which is how long this process of full executive skills development in the brain takes.

In the course of development, our brain and nervous system, in conjunction with our body, provide us with an ever-increasing capacity to move about in our environment, interact with it, and receive feedback about that interaction. It is in the context of these interactions with the world that executive skills develop. When we practice crossing the street with our 6-year-old, holding her hand and telling her, "Stop, look both ways," that experience becomes encoded in the neurobiological substrate of our child's brain. Over time, we can fade the hand holding, and eventually even the words, as we see evidence that our child is learning the skill and demonstrating safety by using memory, inhibition, and attention.

Over the course of 25 years, your child's accumulation of these types of skills through practice strengthens the capacity for the self-regulation that depends on executive skills. The child's interaction with *people* (parents, teachers, community members, and peers) and with *things* (phones, cars, ATMs, washers and dryers) becomes part of the learning process. And if the process goes as planned, the end result is that your child is more able to make his own decisions and manage for himself and needs to rely less and less on you. If, on the other hand, your young adult is stuck, chances are that a weakness in executive skills has interrupted the process.

Executive Skills Development in Young Adults

Young adults, at least in the United States, are "legal" at age 21, that is, able to buy alcohol and in some states marijuana. But we often think of adulthood beginning at age 18, because that's when many privileges and responsibilities are acquired, and many leave home for college at that age too. Whether your adult child is stalled at age 18, 21, or beyond, however, you're probably providing ongoing advice along with emotional and material support, because you recognize that the parenting role is not defined completely by your child's age. In fact, parenting a young adult is one of the most important phases of your role. Your help and support during the young adult years serve as the launch point and final step of the process you've been preparing your child for since birth— independence from you.

Two facts about young adults justify your ongoing support and need to be taken into account when you carefully consider how to manage this later stage of your parenting role.

1. At least through the mid-20s, executive skills are still developing. That means young adults, particularly those who haven't launched, may need continued support with some of these skills. Identifying a young adult's executive skills strengths as well as those that lag behind becomes a key issue for goal selection and goal achievement. If a young adult chooses a goal based on interest but attaining that goal requires a set of executive skills that are weak, the goal may be a questionable fit. Jackson wants to complete school, but he struggles with task initiation and sustained attention. While this doesn't preclude school completion, he will need some effective strategies to address these weaknesses if he is to succeed.

Colin recalls the error in metacognition—one of the last executive skills to develop and the one through which we see the big picture of a situation accurately and learn from experience —that led him on a fruitless course in AP physics:

> There was also a mental math that was the little voice in my head; it was always there and still is. "Your grades in other courses were okay. More important, you had 2½ years of A's and B's padding your GPA; taking this hit wouldn't do much to it. It will be seen as a fluke, as a case of senioritis. At this point, in terms of stress and time commitment, you're better off chalking it up as an acceptable loss and moving on." So that's what I did. I hung on to a D in the class and scored a 1 on the AP test . And in a way I was right; it barely nudged my GPA, and it was perceived as a case of someone who wasn't a "math" person getting in over his head. Now, partly that was true, but it also revealed my lack of foresight, as so many college courses are built on the format of an initial, familiarizing survey, followed by a rapid incline. And it was the first instance of a pattern of behavior that I would repeat many times in the future.

2. Many young adults have not had a lot of practice with the skills of independent living. At a basic level, these skills include grocery shopping, use of washers and dryers, résumés and job searches, and getting to work on time. At a more advanced level, they include locating apartments and handling leases, and managing money, independent living expenses and budgets, credit, health and car insurance, car repairs, and medical appointments.

Our role as parents is not to manage these areas for our young adults. Nor is it to direct them, in a step-by-step teaching or lecturing fashion, in what they should do. Rather, it is to model these skills for them by inviting them to see, ask questions about, and participate in the ways that we manage these activities for ourselves. We share our tools with them (e.g., budgeting software programs or tricks we've learned for managing our time so we're not late to work). We also may put them in touch with people in the community who can provide these services for them—doctors, dentists, bankers, insurance brokers, or online services that we currently use and they will need—so that they can develop some facility in managing their own affairs.

In so doing, we are, in a sense, killing two birds with one stone. As we've noted, brain development in the regions tied to executive skills continues into young adulthood. So this is the ideal time for young adults to work on these skills. The complex activities of daily living we're talking about are the foundation of our ability to live independently, and mastery of these activities requires executive skills. As our young adults are learning the skills they need to be independent, the practice involved in learning these skills helps them "beef up" the executive skills needed for other life goals. Furthermore, how young adults manage these activities gives us direct evidence about their executive skills strengths and weaknesses and what supports they may need to strengthen their skill set. In fact, you may discover executive skills weaknesses that weren't as evident at home or school once the young adult is expected to handle daily adult tasks for the first time. We offer practical advice for helping young adults develop these skills of independent living in the Appendix.

The Essential Dozen: Definitions of the Executive Skills Needed for Independence and Success

Let's drill down a bit and identify the specific executive skills we believe are at the core of independent adulthood. Neuroscientists organize and label executive skills in different ways, and in fact some even call them executive *functions*. We prefer to use the word *skills* because we know that these are behaviors that can be learned and practiced. And by so doing, we can become more proficient at them, in the same way a tennis player practicing serves or volleys day in and day out gets better at playing tennis. To us, the word *function* sounds more permanent and less malleable—like brakes on a car. They're there and they function to stop the car to avoid hitting something. We're much more interested in the *skill* involved in learning how to use the braking function proficiently.

We began our work on executive skills by identifying the skills we thought were critical to school success. We very quickly realized that the same skills predicted adult success as well. And through the years we've found that our terminology helps people visualize and operationalize the skills. You may find more technical descriptions of executive skills out there, but we place a premium on clarity.

The definitions and brief behavioral examples in the checklist on pages 27–29 are designed to introduce executive skills and a sample of the behaviors that exemplify these skills. You and your young adult can read through this list, and if you find the examples of each skill helpful in describing how you each see yourself, you can enter your initials on that line. (The checklist is also available online; see the end of the Contents for information.) A more complete assessment questionnaire for the young adult follows on pages 31–33. Parents can assess their own executive skills more fully in Step 4.

What can you take from these definitions? Getting an idea of where your young adult's executive skills and weaknesses may lie? What about your own?

Assessing the Young Adult's Executive Skills

As we already mentioned, Jackson really does want to further his education. The courses he's taking online will get him some credits toward a degree in environmental science. And he's really interested in environmental engineering. But he's not going to get into that highly competitive field unless he actually gets the degree. Terry doesn't like living at home with her parents. She got pretty used to coming and going as she pleased when she was living and working at a resort over the summer and then into the fall, but the off-season didn't pay enough for her to live on her own once her roommate went back to college. Unfortunately, her job search from home has gone through fits and starts, and 3 months later she's still unemployed. Tirone's having lost several jobs due to being disorganized is eroding his self-confidence, which he tries to hide from his parents with gruff silence—which they're interpreting as his lack of concern about paying them back when he actually feels really guilty about that but doesn't know how to resolve his problems.

All three of these young adults have a broad goal—get a job, get a degree, make enough money to repay parents—but no idea about how to reach it. A good start is to take a close look at what's holding them back. Is the broad goal too broad? Is it realistic? Will it be met, considering the individual's executive skills profile?

Executive Skills Definitions and Behaviors Checklist

Check off or initial behaviors/statements that you identify with.

Response Inhibition: The capacity to think before you act—this ability to resist the urge to say or do something allows us the time to evaluate a situation and how our behavior might impact it.

Strong	Weak
_____ Thinks before speaking	_____ Says first thing thought of
_____ "It's worth waiting for"	_____ "I want it now"
_____ Reflects on decisions	_____ Makes impulsive decisions

Working Memory: The ability to hold information in memory while performing complex tasks. It incorporates the ability to draw on past learning or experience to apply to the situation at hand or to project into the future.

Strong	Weak
_____ Keeps track of belongings	_____ Misplaces things
_____ Remembers what to do	_____ "What was I going to do?"
_____ Learns from past experience	_____ Repeats same mistakes

Emotional Control: The ability to manage emotions in order to achieve goals, complete tasks, or control and direct behavior.

Strong	Weak
_____ Maintains cool	_____ Has a short fuse
_____ Handles criticism/correction	_____ Is easily hurt/aggravated
_____ Controls temper if frustrated	_____ Tends to "lose it" if frustrated

Task Initiation: The ability to begin projects without undue procrastination, in an efficient or timely fashion.

Strong	Weak
_____ Gets started right away	_____ Dawdles
_____ "Just do it"	_____ "Plenty of time"
_____ "I took care of it"	_____ "I promise I'll take care of it"

(continued)

Sustained Attention: The capacity to maintain attention to a situation or task in spite of distractibility, fatigue, or boredom.

Strong	Weak
_____ Finishes the task	_____ Jumps around
_____ Persists at job	_____ "This is boring"
_____ Focused	_____ Easily distracted

Planning/Prioritization: The ability to create a road map to reach a goal or to complete a task. It also involves being able to make decisions about what's important to focus on and what's not important.

Strong	Weak
_____ Sees path to the goal	_____ Not sure how to get there
_____ "This is the first thing to do"	_____ "Start here, no, maybe there?"
_____ "I can ignore this"	_____ "Is this important?"

Organization: The ability to create and maintain systems to keep track of information or materials.

Strong	Weak
_____ Neat, tidy	_____ Stuff everywhere
_____ A place for everything	_____ Wherever it fits
_____ "It's right here"	_____ "I don't know where it is"

Time Management: The capacity to estimate how much time one has, how to allocate it, and how to stay within time limits and deadlines. It also involves a sense that time is important.

Strong	Weak
_____ "This will take 10 minutes"	_____ "This will take forever"
_____ "I need to leave now"	_____ "Just one more thing before I go"
_____ "It's due today"	_____ "An extra day is no big deal"

(continued)

Goal-Directed Persistence: The capacity to have a goal, to follow through to the completion of the goal, and to not be put off by or distracted by competing interests.

Strong	Weak
_____ "Come hell or high water"	_____ "This is too much work"
_____ "It's worth the wait"	_____ "I want it now"
_____ "I can get past this"	_____ "I'll never get past this"

Flexibility: The ability to revise plans in the face of obstacles, setbacks, new information, or mistakes. It relates to an adaptability to changing conditions.

Strong	Weak
_____ Go with the flow	_____ Stick to the schedule
_____ "Maybe there's another way"	_____ "There's only one way"
_____ Spontaneous	_____ Set in ways

Metacognition: The ability to stand back and take a bird's-eye view of oneself in a situation. It is an ability to observe how you problem-solve. It also includes self-monitoring and self-evaluative skills (e.g., asking yourself "How am I doing?" or "How did I do?").

Strong	Weak
_____ "I'm okay at this"	_____ "Am I any good at this?"
_____ "I'd give myself a B"	_____ "How did I do?"
_____ "This relates to this"	_____ "I don't see any connection"

Stress Tolerance: The ability to thrive in stressful situations and to cope with uncertainty, change, and performance demands.

Strong	Weak
_____ Take it in stride	_____ Overwhelmed
_____ "I can manage this"	_____ "I can't do it"
_____ "Let's see what happens"	_____ "I need to know exactly what is happening"

Young adults should fill out the questionnaire on pages 31–33 (also available online; see the end of the Contents for information) so they can start to see whether there is a good fit between where they want to go and what executive skills they have to get there.

Any surprises here? Does this information explain what has been holding the young adult back? Where have you seen the executive skills weaknesses cause problems with momentum? Where have strengths been helpful? Many parents and young adults find the results of the questionnaire a relief. Finally, they have an idea of why it's been hard to get going or to keep going. A young adult who doesn't tolerate stress well might not do well in an intensive 4-year degree program right away but thrive at a community college where success can be built one or two courses at a time. An adult child who is relatively low in response inhibition and task initiation won't be likely to succeed in a job that calls for disciplined self-starters. Someone who doesn't have time management or planning skills may flounder when simply expected to "go out and get a job." He won't know where—or when or how—to start and will need more support from you.

> As a favor to Peg and my dad, I did fill out the Executive Skills Questionnaire toward the end of high school. I don't remember exactly my profile, but I'd guess strengths would have been flexibility and stress tolerance. Weaknesses are clearer—task initiation, sustained attention, and goal-directed persistence [GDP]. In the spring of this year, 2017, it's a bit different. I see my strengths now as flexibility, metacognition, and emotional control. Task initiation and sustained attention persist as weaknesses, and time management has moved into third place (from fourth in the past). Having a career objective that has emerged clearly only in the past 3 years has helped displace GDP as a weakness.

Colin's profiles, then and now, are not a surprise to me or my wife. What is or was surprising is that with my own son I didn't attend to and act on what I knew. For any other teen with this executive skills profile and his or her parents I would have predicted the likely outcome and the steps they could take to avoid it. Colin even gave us his vision of what was to come. On an evening a few weeks before we took him to college, my wife and I were talking with him about last-minute details. In the midst of the conversation, very uncharacteristic for him, he broke down, saying he didn't think he could succeed. I chalked

Executive Skills Questionnaire

Read each item below and then rate that item based on the extent to which you agree or disagree with how well it describes you. Use the rating scale below to choose the appropriate score. Then add the three scores in each section. Use the Key at the end of the questionnaire to determine your executive skills strengths (two or three highest scores) and weaknesses (two or three lowest scores). Everyone who completes this questionnaire will have some strengths and some weaknesses. No pattern of strengths or weaknesses is "better" or "worse" than any other, and there is no pattern that is "typical" or "atypical."

Strongly disagree	1	Tend to agree	4
Disagree	2	Agree	5
Tend to disagree	3	Strongly agree	6

Item   **Your score**

1. I don't jump to conclusions. _____

2. I think before I speak. _____

3. I make sure I have all the facts before I take action. _____

           TOTAL _____

4. I have a good memory for facts, dates, and details. _____

5. I am very good at remembering the things I have committed to do. _____

6. I seldom need reminders to complete tasks. _____

           TOTAL _____

7. My emotions seldom get in the way when performing on the job. _____

8. Little things do not affect me emotionally or distract me from the task at hand. _____

9. When frustrated or angry, I keep my cool. _____

           TOTAL _____

10. No matter what the task, I believe in getting started as soon as possible. _____

11. Procrastination is usually not a problem for me. _____

12. I seldom leave tasks to the last minute. _____

           TOTAL _____

(continued)

Item	Your score
13. I find it easy to stay focused on my work.	_____
14. Once I start an assignment, I work diligently until it's completed.	_____
15. Even when interrupted, I find it easy to get back and complete the job at hand.	_____
TOTAL	_____
16. When I start my day, I have a clear plan in mind for what I hope to accomplish.	_____
17. When I have a lot to do, I can easily focus on the most important things.	_____
18. I typically break big tasks down into subtasks and timelines.	_____
TOTAL	_____
19. I am an organized person.	_____
20. It is natural for me to keep my work area neat and organized.	_____
21. I am good at maintaining systems for organizing my work.	_____
TOTAL	_____
22. At the end of the day, I've usually finished what I set out to do.	_____
23. I am good at estimating how long it takes to do something.	_____
24. I am usually on time for appointments and activities.	_____
TOTAL	_____
25. I take unexpected events in stride.	_____
26. I easily adjust to changes in plans and priorities.	_____
27. I consider myself to be flexible and adaptive to change.	_____
TOTAL	_____
28. I routinely evaluate my performance and devise methods for personal improvement.	_____
29. I am able to step back from a situation in order to make objective decisions.	_____
30. I am a "big picture" thinker and enjoy the problem solving that goes with that.	_____
TOTAL	_____

(continued)

Item	Your score
31. I think of myself as being driven to meet my goals.	_____
32. I easily give up immediate pleasures to work on long-term goals.	_____
33. I believe in setting and achieving high levels of performance.	_____
	TOTAL _____
34. I enjoy working in a highly demanding, fast-paced environment.	_____
35. A certain amount of pressure helps me to perform at my best.	_____
36. Jobs that include a fair degree of unpredictability appeal to me.	_____
	TOTAL _____

KEY

Items	Executive skill	Items	Executive skill
1–3	Response inhibition	4–6	Working memory
7–9	Emotional control	10–12	Task initiation
13–15	Sustained attention	16–18	Planning/prioritization
19–21	Organization	22–24	Time management
25–27	Flexibility	28–30	Metacognition
31–33	Goal-directed persistence	34–36	Stress tolerance

Strongest Skills (highest scores)   **Weakest Skills (lowest scores)**

_____   _____

_____   _____

_____   _____

What Did You Learn?

What did the questionnaire tell you are the young adult's two or three strongest executive skills and two or three weakest skills? Enter them below for easy reference if you like.

Executive Skills Strengths

_____

_____

Executive Skills Weaknesses

_____

_____

it up to last-minute stress and reassured him and my wife that he'd be fine. It was a wake-up call and a lesson that I haven't forgotten. I came to know that he is the best judge of what's best for him. (He was probably already becoming strong in metacognition!) Over time I've become a better listener, and he, in turn, openly discusses problems and doubts and we discuss options. He chooses which, if any, makes sense for him and when he wants help. He's open to suggestions and knows for himself what fits best. And I've learned to listen and to appreciate collaborative problem solving. I've given a specific example below.

So what do you do with your list of executive skills weaknesses and strengths? We're going to show you how to consider the implications in setting good goals toward achieving independence in the next few steps. But later in the book—in Steps 7 and 8—we'll also show you how you can adapt the tasks and environments of adult life to an individual's executive skills profile and also how young adults can get creative, as Colin and many others have, to compensate for specific executive skills deficits.

The Collaboration Begins

Now is a good time to start collaborating, so we encourage parents and young adults to sit down and talk about the questionnaire results and any insights they produce. For Colin and me, our collaboration began in earnest when he decided in 2014, 9 years after graduating from high school, that he needed a college degree to pursue his interest in behavior analysis and autism. Now he had a goal, but he recognized that the executive skills weaknesses were likely to be an impediment, especially since he would have to take courses that were not relevant to his interests. These had always been his Achilles' heel. Ability was never the issue. Rather, it was on-time completion of tedious work. We discussed how I might help, and he proposed that I prompt him and follow his progress with on-time completion of coursework. And so we embarked on a process that, with fits and starts, stretched out over 2 years. And it continues, in a much-reduced form today, in late 2017. Colin is pursuing a master's degree in behavioral psychology. If he feels stuck and has questions, say for a research paper, he calls or texts and we talk through his thoughts. Since we share an interest in behavior analysis, our collaboration typically involves confirmation that his approach makes sense and that is enough for him to move on.

To compound the problem of executive skills challenges, many young adults who have been experiencing disappointments in pursuing higher education, getting a job, or doing much of anything independently can find themselves increasingly demoralized or even depressed. Their motivation and self-confidence often take a serious hit. If you've been thinking your son or daughter "just isn't motivated," you might be right, but not due to an underlying character flaw. Here's Colin's memory of his experience.

> I think when I got to the later parts of high school and the beginning of college, I wasn't used to there having to be a real embodiment of hard work or focus in order to achieve. I understood what people meant when they said work hard, give 110%, and study, but for most of the time I didn't have to internalize that message, even though the results indicated I did. And when the time came for me to understand that I was no longer smart enough to get A's and B's on autopilot, I didn't want or really know how to do things differently.
>
> I was like a young kid who was really good at basketball because I liked shooting around in my free time. And when people saw me play they thought, wow, he's going to be really good someday. But I wasn't really good then because I desperately wanted to play in college or the NBA. I was just good as a kid because I liked playing and was a little bit taller than everyone else. Then one day I'm in high school and people are telling me to watch game film, and two-a-day practices, and suicides [increasingly longer, timed sprints, with a change in direction for each sprint] till you puke. And I thought playing in college must be a good idea because all my teammates were busting their butts to get recruited. But I was angry and resentful that my old moves didn't really work anymore, and when I got to college the coach told me what it would take to be a starter, and I said, eh, things will work out. And then I got outplayed and got frustrated and didn't know how to adjust my game or whether it was really "my sport" in the first place. Similar experiences in arenas of my life were just as frustrating, and they ate away at my self-confidence and my motivation to get involved in new endeavors.

Launching into adult life is a complicated process for some postadolescents. Some problems involved reside in the young adult individually, such as executive skills deficits or a lack of awareness of what the young adult wants to do and has the talent or aptitude to take on. Some reside in the parent individually—unrealistic expectations, the parent's own executive skills, or the parent's attitudes about independence and providing support toward it. Some have to do with the dynamics between parent and adult child. If there's nothing you love more than making lists and plans and checking off met objectives, but the preceding questionnaire shows that your child lacks planning skills, you two may have been clashing for years. If you tell your son you want him to find his dream future but then you subtly take the helm over and over to steer him toward *your* dream, you could be giving mixed messages that paralyze him. If you say your daughter really needs to take responsibility for her own upkeep but then you keep doing her laundry and waking her up for work, you're not really giving her the opportunity to take care of herself.

Knowing the young adult's executive skills profile can help you defuse blame and guilt by pointing to concrete reasons it may have been tough for the young adult to move toward independence. It may explain why progress has not been made toward any goal the young adult has set—or why no goal has been set at all. For a goal to be achievable, it has to meet the criteria for goodness of fit: Is the goal a good fit with the young adult's executive skills? Is the goal a good fit for what the adult child wants and has the talent or aptitude to do? To identify a desirable and realistic goal, both you and the young adult also need to be motivated to collaborate on it. Are you both ready? The next chapter, Step 2, will help you see where you two stand on readiness for change and motivation. Then you can get to know yourselves better individually in Steps 3 and 4— young adults getting to know in detail what they want and what skills, talents, and knowledge they can apply to it; and parents digging in to discover how they really feel about their children leaving the nest and what they're willing to contribute over the long haul to support the child's pursuit of independence.

STEP 2

....

Build a Foundation for Moving Forward
Motivation, Readiness, Respect, and Support

"Hey, Jonas, I got an e-mail from your aunt and uncle; they're gonna be traveling through here in a couple of weeks and would like to get together for dinner. Are you good with that?"

"Yeah, of course. They don't need my okay."

"No, I mean can you join us?"

"Ahh, yeah I guess, if nothing comes up."

"Umm, a bit more definite?"

"Sure, okay . . . Wait, is this gonna be some kinda third degree about my future?"

"Where'd that come from?"

"They've asked before."

"Relax, they like you, and I'd hardly call 'Have you thought about what you'd like for work?' the third degree."

"Mom, we've been here, I like my job, I like my life, end of story."

"J, you're in a low-paying job, you're living at home, and if there's a plan on the horizon, I haven't been clued in. . . . Is there a plan?"

"I can't do this, I gotta go, talk to you later."

Young adults like Jonas baffle their parents. Here's a bright, healthy, 22-year-old with a supportive family who had a fairly comfortable childhood. He has the social skills to have made friends all his life. He can make conversation with his parents' generation and young children as well as with his peers. He seems to keep himself pretty well entertained, rather than dragging himself around as if his feet are stuck in the mud like the kids described by some of his parents' friends.

Yet there's no doubt that Jonas is stuck. He can't figure out an educational or career direction and hasn't budged toward leaving home. Taking the Executive Skills Questionnaire in Step 1 has helped Jonas and his parents understand some of what is holding him back. He has weaknesses in task initiation, sustained attention, and time management, which explains a lot of his difficulties in sticking with college.

But it still doesn't seem to explain everything. Jonas generally liked school and got involved in various hobbies and activities over his childhood. Nothing really lasted, but he wasn't one of those kids who did nothing but watch TV, surf the Internet, or play video games. So why, his parents keep asking each other, is he still wandering aimlessly when they've watched "everyone else" go off to college, graduate, and find a job and a place to live?

Jonas's parents' comparisons of their son with his peers are, of course, based on incomplete information. They don't have any idea how much support other kids' parents had to provide, the wrangling that went on over a child's decisions, the failures and disappointments that disrupted progress. This didn't stop them from lamenting the fact that *their* child is the "only one" who hasn't kept pace.

The fact is that getting any teenager on track toward an independent future is a complicated process that requires fortitude, patience, understanding, and support. The path is undeniably clearer if the child has a good set of executive skills. But even for a child with few executive skills deficiencies (although all of us have comparative strengths and weaknesses), other factors come into play. One significant factor is motivation: Does your son or daughter *want* to become independent? Another is readiness for change: Is he or she prepared to take steps toward independence or is he or she really adrift?

Lest you believe only the young adult's motivation and readiness for change matter, know that *your* motivation and readiness should be considered too—and your influence over your child's motivation and readiness. What is your attitude toward independence? Are *you* truly ready for your son or daughter to leave home? Mixed messages on this issue from you could be leading your child to seem unmotivated when he's really trying to figure out what you want and provide it. What do you picture your adult child doing as an adult? Do you know whether it's what she pictures doing—or wants to do? If the young adult doesn't seem very ready to change, is it possible that he or she needs some kind of collaboration with you that he or she can't really describe and doesn't know how to ask for?

Collaboration starts with clear, calm communication about expectations and definition of roles. At this step, we'll give you food for thought about what independence might mean to each of you, who should be making decisions, the importance of motivation and how to boost it, and the essential groundwork of readiness for change. Let's start with independence. If you two can't agree on what that destination means, it will be difficult to establish goals and objectives to help the young adult reach it.

What Do You Mean by "Independence"?

The first and probably most frequent hurdle that parents face in moving ahead and supporting their young adult is a willingness to abide by a relatively simple definition of independence. It may seem obvious to you, but there are degrees and stages of independence, and it's important to know what you and your adult child are expecting. Complete self-sufficiency? Living at home but working and making financial contributions to the household? Simply starting to do his own laundry and cooking and looking for a job? Is there a timeline?

Independence can take shape in different ways depending on your family circumstances, but we've found that the most effective foundation for progress is this simple definition:

If the goal or subgoal that your young adult arrives at in Step 5 results in a greater level of self-sufficiency than she has in her present situation and offers the opportunity for additional change and additional self-sufficiency, it meets the criteria for becoming independent—even though independence will probably be reached somewhat gradually.

Your son or daughter may have a goal right now. If so, does it seem to meet these criteria? If the goal is to go away to college, that demands that the child become more self-sufficient than she's been while living at home. If she succeeds there, she'll be more prepared for additional self-sufficiency armed with a degree, which might lead to a job on a particular career path. Therefore, the goal meets our criteria. But what if she doesn't succeed at college?

I remember sitting with Colin in a presentation for incoming students and their parents given by the college counseling center at the beginning of Colin's freshman year. They talked about the dangers of alcohol and drugs, unprotected sex, and the need for students to step up and be "responsible" for themselves. And to the adults accompanying their children, they spoke about the dangers of being a "helicopter" parent who meddles in the life of the child when that "child" is learning to be on his own. They said not a word about executive skills, nor gave any indication they had ever heard of the concept. I do remember thinking that they were naïve about the transition process, and that a factor they seemed unaware of likely accounted for a sizable number of students who would flunk out during their freshman year. I just didn't think about Colin in that calculation.

Over the next two and a half years, "helicopter" label be damned, we tried to put into place some semblance of what we had done in high school and what Colin would tolerate. Colin had also stepped up from day one of college to either use whatever money he had of his own or take out loans to pay for school, and my wife and I agreed to pay his tuition at the state university for the courses he passed. He found some courses he liked and had some, but for him not sufficient, success, and he told us at what would have been the beginning of his junior year that he thought it would be better to stay in a job he had started that summer rather than return to school. That's when he decided to stay on the island, which turned out to be a valuable experience for him even if it didn't fulfill our dream for him.

> My landscaping job provided the structural middle ground between home and college. A job isn't something your parents will make sure you go to every day; they won't talk to your boss about your performance and have talks with you about it at dinner (at least not typically; I'm sure there are situations when this happens—bear with me). But you'll lose your job if you don't show up for work, and your coworkers will have to do your work for you. My job started as something I couldn't lose because I had nothing else, but it became more about doing my share for the company and not saddling my peers (who were also friends) with the load that created a sense of responsibility. In college, if I was failing, no one else failed, and professors weren't supposed to piggyback me the whole way through the course. I didn't understand at the time that even in college, with no structure, my parents and friends were my coworkers in an abstract way. I don't mean that everyone pastes pictures of their family on their notebooks to constantly remind them why they're there. And I'm not saying I think other people are running around with motivational poster epithets blaring in their heads. People don't always consciously think about why they go to college, but most of them go because they have some general idea of how things are supposed to look in their lives, or they grew up in an environment where that process was assumed, counted on, even if it was implicit. It may sound strange, but that is

a concept that never materialized in my mind until well after I left college.

What work did for me is teach me that even though adults are "independent," independent is a word that can never include all of its meanings at once. It's freedom to choose but not be independent of the consequences.

Colin's experience demonstrates an important possibility: the goal may meet our criteria for independence but not be achievable at this stage in the young adult's life. This could be due to executive skills deficiencies—as was true for Colin, and I suspect is the case with many students who boomerang back home after an initial shot at college. Colin wasn't fully prepared for the independence of college, and he wasn't all that motivated to put in the effort he would have needed to exert to do well. This may be because motivation and readiness feed on each other, for good or ill. A young adult who aims for a goal that requires executive skills he doesn't have is bound to feel discouraged by a lack of success. One who learns ways to compensate for weak skills (as described in Steps 7 and 8), and as a result experiences some success, is going to feel motivated to keep going. As Colin just described, he was in some ways more prepared for the independence of living away from home and holding down a job than for the independence associated with college, partly because of the divergent skill requirements of a job versus college.

This may not be true for your young adult, however. In Step 1 we urged you to remember that many young adults don't have much experience with the basic skills of independent living, from doing their own laundry to acquiring car insurance. They're no more prepared for living away from home and getting to a job every day than they are for getting a bachelor's degree. When you're focused on an educational and occupational path toward independence for your young adult, the need to learn how to perform daily adult functions can slip down your priority list. But as you can see, our definition of independence encompasses these types of goals as well as getting a degree or a job, because they too will lead to further independence. How to define independence for a specific young adult depends on the individual's starting point.

> *Independence means different things in different settings and to different people.*

Have you asked your young adult how he defines independence? You might be surprised that he doesn't really know, possibly because the mere thought of taking care of himself overwhelms him. This could be the case if your young adult has already bounced back from college or is so stuck that he has no idea

what to do with his days now that he is out of high school and he is still depending on you to support him financially, feed him, and make his car payments.

Many parents think of college, because it does *not* impose all the demands
of a truly self-sufficient life, as a transitional step between childhood and adulthood. They assume, therefore, that college independence will be easier to handle than sending a child out into the job world and expecting him to support
himself. What about your son or daughter? If your son can't handle the academic
pressures of college, could he do better in a job he has the essential skills to do?
If your daughter can't resist the temptation to break all of your house rules now
that she's not living under your roof, would she do better living back at home
and going to community college for a while? Or getting a job, living at home,
and saving her own money for tuition before trying to go away to college again?

These are all questions to mull over as you and your young adult consider
where she is right now, where you both want her to go, how long it should
take to get her there, and what goals and objectives need to be set to arrive at
independence. It really is important, however, not to skip the step of determin-
ing what you both envision when you think about the term "independent."
Yes, it should fit the criteria laid out earlier and at its core involve greater self-
sufficiency than currently exists. But what does this mean in real-world terms
for the two of you, as you view it right now? Use the checklist on page 43 as a
starting point for your discussions. Any discrepancies between you two need to
be discussed, probably on an ongoing basis, so that you both have your eye on
the same destination. In fact, you should probably revisit this checklist periodically, since the current baseline of self-sufficiency will evolve and therefore the
elements of increasing independence will too (the checklist is also available
online; see the end of the Contents for information).

What Does This Transition Mean for the Young Adult and the Parent?

If your discussion of what independence really means reveals some disagreements, why do you think they exist? Maybe one of you is overconfident about
the young adult's abilities and readiness for change. Maybe one or both of you
has been bruised by previous disappointments in the trek toward independence
and fears repeating the same mistakes. A young adult who is ambivalent or
even resistant about moving ahead toward independence may be feeling pretty
anxious. Any history of failing to achieve a goal or disappointing adult expectations is likely to plant doubts in the young adult's mind about whether he'll be

How Do You Two Define Independence?

What's included in your definition?

Parent	Young Adult	
☐	☐	No financial support from parents (Ps)
☐	☐	Less financial support from Ps
☐	☐	Young adult (YA) living in and paying for separate residence
☐	☐	YA living separately but receiving rent subsidy from Ps
☐	☐	YA living at home and paying rent
☐	☐	YA living at home for free but helping with chores, etc.
☐	☐	YA living at home for free, not helping out
☐	☐	YA living at home, handling own cooking, laundry, etc.
☐	☐	YA having a job and saving money for own education
☐	☐	Ps paying tuition on condition of agreed-on level of academic success
☐	☐	YA has a part-time job and goes to school part-time
☐	☐	YA has a full-time job
☐	☐	YA has a full-time job with career potential
☐	☐	YA lives by his/her own rules while living at home
☐	☐	YA follows Ps' rules if receiving any financial support
☐	☐	YA adheres to same rules at home as when under age 18
☐	☐	Independence should start immediately
☐	☐	Independence should be achieved within an agreed-on time period
☐	☐	Independence should occur gradually, without pressure of deadlines

successful. Moving away from dependence on parents may feel like walking into the unknown, not knowing what's coming or how to get there and at the same time realizing that the safety net that parents have provided throughout life is at least receding into the distance. And even if the safety net remains available to some degree, there may be ambivalence about using it because there may be strings attached and they can undermine the sense of independence.

Are You Ready to Let Go?

There can also be ambivalence about change from parents. Parents can feel concern or anxiety about the young adult's ability to manage responsibility and independence based on their typically long-standing desire to protect their children from major disappointment or harm. And who among us hasn't felt that the young adult doesn't really understand what it takes to transition to successful adult living? This feeling is especially likely if your young adult has stalled and you're watching her struggle in this transition. In addition, we are a generation of parents who are involved with our children's lives in a way that our parents probably were not. That means that we've taken a more active role in their lives both at school and in their extracurricular activities—music, the arts, and sports. If, by virtue of stalling, they've stayed at home or have moved back home or in some fashion remain financially tied to us, we continue to remain active in their lives.

For some parents, the transition of the young adult from dependent to more independent can trigger a sense of loss, both of time spent with the child and in terms of caretaking and giving us a sense of purpose. We use terms like "empty-nest syndrome." And while our children will still come to us for advice and support, we will not occupy the primary position as advisor that we had in the past. If you were envisioning a newfound freedom with your child's exit from the nest and he's still in it, you may feel frustrated by the inability to pursue your own dreams. Given your young adult's simultaneous need for support and demand for freedom in the context of living at home, this can feel like taxation without representation.

These are real and legitimate feelings for parents and young adults that arise out of the life transition of dependent childhood to independent adulthood. When young adults are halted in this transition, what would have been a naturally occurring final stage of childhood development stops and leads to frustration and stress. If both parties, in the face of this stress, revert to their respective roles of parent and child, the transition process will remain slowed and the paralysis may deepen. When young adults are stuck and struggling, parents are much more likely to turn to the parental role with which they are familiar and young adults are more likely to return to the primary support system that throughout their life has provided them with assistance and comfort. The one factor that legislates against this state of affairs is that both parties return to their familiar roles with some ambivalence and hesitation, knowing (hopefully) that this cannot go on indefinitely.

Whose Future Is It?

Even if the ultimate goal is longer term, a young adult's anxiety makes it essential that young adults and parents focus on very short and concrete accomplishments or objectives with little or no focus on the long-term goal. This can be a hard undertaking for parents. Like most parents, you probably have had and continue to have some hopes and dreams for your child. If you know from your child's history and experiences that he has interests and abilities, then you very likely have a vision about what he might become or what he might accomplish. If you accept your young adult's goal, then that means that you need to give up, or at least put on indefinite hold, some of your own hopes and dreams for your child. This is especially difficult if the goal you have for your child seems more sensible or "more realistic" than what he is proposing.

> *"Jonas, did you mean what you said about going to school for IT?"*
>
> *Marta poured herself a black coffee while her son ritually reads the classifieds at a stool in the kitchen.*
>
> *"What? When did I say that?"*
>
> *"When your uncle and Julie were over for dinner the other night. They asked about school, and you said you were thinking about IT or 'some kind of tech job' I think was how you described it."*
>
> *"Oh, ha, Mom, that was like 4 days ago. And I don't know, I just said it, you know? It kind of came up in conversation, and I said it. I haven't given it a lot of thought since."*
>
> *"Gotcha. Mmm, yikes, that's hot!" Marta half-dropped the cup on the counter and quickly reached for a paper towel to mop up the sloshing. "I was just curious. I know we've talked a lot, a lot, about what you want to do over the last 8 months or so. I hadn't really heard you say anything about IT before, so when it came up it kind of set off my radar. Does that stuff interest you at all?"*
>
> *"Um, I don't know . . . maybe? I like what I do with computers, but I don't know much about it as a job, and I don't know whether liking something as a hobby is gonna mean I'll like it as a career, you know?"*
>
> *"No, I understand, I get it. You like it, but when you think about doing it for 25 years it doesn't really paint a clear picture for you."*

"Right."

Marta smiled and leaned over toward Jonas, peeling down the corner of the paper so she could see his whole face. "Well, is there anything that does show a clearer picture? You know that I love you and think you should stay here with me until the end of time. On the other hand, it feels like it's been long enough that things are starting to . . . settle, in a way that makes me a little worried. Not that you won't find out what you want to do, but that maybe we aren't figuring that out with as much urgency as you otherwise would. I want you to start again from a place of comfort and stability, but I do want you to start again."

Jonas is stalled, and his mother wants to get him going, so she jumps at any sign of an interest and immediately transforms it into a career path. Yet this approach is almost always doomed to fail. Your approach, possibly even your dream, does not make for the kind of independent (while still collaborative) decision making that cultivates motivation and progress.

> *Jumping to turn an interest into a career path to get a young adult going is bound to fail.*

"But Where Will This Get You in the Long Term?"

There is a second element that is typically part of the goals or hopes that parents have for their child. Most parents hope that their child chooses a path that leads to long-term stability, self-sufficiency, and a secure future. For example, for some parents, graduating from college with a degree that can immediately lead to a career path fulfills this imagined security. Computing, engineering, nursing, teaching, accounting, and some other majors would fulfill this vision. A degree that feeds naturally into graduate or professional school also offers this hoped-for security. For other parents this security might come from a skilled trade—mechanic, cook, chef, plumber, or carpenter. Or perhaps a parent envisions an associate's degree that leads to a path in a particular industry, as is the focus of an increasing number of partnerships between community colleges and businesses. Or maybe you see your daughter's future in one of the armed services. The point is that as parents we do not just want to see independence or self-sufficiency; we want to see it in the context of some type of career that has a future. The young adult's goal may not in any obvious way lead to such security.

> *Be careful not to demand that the young adult's goal have "a future" by your definition.*

When Colin took his job landscaping on the island, his mother and I were happy that he had achieved some stability and independence. At the same time, we were nagged by the question that if this wasn't going to be his long-term career, what was coming next and was there a connection between this job and what would follow it? When the goal is more immediate and may well meet the criteria of independence we've defined, the lack of more certainty about the long term can be unsettling and anxiety-provoking for the parents. This leads to both career- and non-career-related questions:

- Does the job have a future?
- With this job will he be able to afford health or car insurance?
- Will he find a partner?

Sound familiar? Maybe you've been greeted by these questions at 2:00 A.M. When adult children reach these types of milestones, parents typically feel pride and a sense that the future is now secure. But if your young adult is struggling to become more independent, accepting her plan and goals often means accepting and living with doubts that you have about her ability to manage responsibility and persist toward a goal. Your thoughts are likely based on past evidence of the young adult seeming to commit to a goal and with good intentions to pursue it only to falter or fail when the task has become effortful. In fact, it may well have been your goal that the young adult initially signed on for and ultimately failed to achieve. That's why, even though from your perspective the goal that you have for your child may seem more sensible and guarantees a more stable future, the fact that he has failed at it is exactly the reason for not revisiting it now and likely plays a role in the young adult's hesitation to undertake and commit to a goal that will take a long time to achieve. If your young adult does choose a goal that involves a longer-term commitment such as moving into one of the skilled professions or obtaining a degree, keep in mind that it is still the achievement of short-term objectives and subgoals that will determine his success. So when you say that you're ready to sign on to your young adult's goal and accept his pursuit plan, keep in mind that you're setting aside some of your own significant concerns and that this can be a struggle.

Colin felt his nearly 2 years on the island was transformative, as it was for my wife and me. He had managed completely on his own, and we realized, and perhaps more importantly accepted, that he could make a life for himself; it seemed he was pretty happy with doing something that was unrelated to what we had thought was the goal that we had all signed on for: finish school in 4 years, get a job, and get on the path to some career. So for us, the new reality was that whatever he wanted to do, as long as he was reasonably happy with it and able to manage his life, was okay.

The Choice Belongs to the Young Adult

We can't stress this point too much. It's your young adult's life, your young adult's future, and so *decisions about goals toward independence have to be based on her dreams, her approach.*

There are two essential reasons the young adult must be in charge of setting her own direction:

1. **Interfering with the young adult's decision-making process or insisting that she follow a path that you prefer makes her dependent.** This moves you back into the parent role that you played earlier in her development.

2. **A person who chooses her own direction or sets her own goal is more likely to be motivated to achieve that goal than if she is doing someone else's bidding.** Research has confirmed this truth, and we've seen it again and again in our coaching.

The take-home message here is that if you want your young adult to move toward independence, you have to make sure you are not explicitly or implicitly encouraging her to remain dependent on you by taking over the decision-making role. You can inadvertently keep your child dependent in a number of ways, by dampening motivation or providing too much or too little support, which we'll discuss below. For now, ask yourself if you can adopt the mindset that will allow you to pass the baton:

- Can you and your young adult agree on a definition of—and timeline for—independence?
- Can you ask the young adult, in a way that invites a candid response, whether the goal he has been pursuing with your approval is the goal he would pursue if allowed to choose freely for himself?
- Can you start a dialogue on what dreams the young adult has and listen with an open ear (and often a closed mouth)?
- Are you willing to consider your young adult's choice of a goal, short or long term, as long as it meets the criteria for independence?

That last question is somewhat premature. You need information you'll gather in Step 3 to determine how realistic any goal may be, but you also need to get a preliminary idea of what types of support you're willing to provide so that your young adult doesn't end up set up for failure (by himself, by you, or with help from both of you!).

What Kind of Support Are You Willing and Able to Offer?

At the end of the almost 2 years on the island, Colin came back feeling that he needed a change and moved in with us for what was intended to be a few months while he job-hunted and planned to move to Boston with a friend. But his friend could never quite seem to get it together—he also was living at home and working for his father—and so the few months stretched into a year. Colin found some part-time work as a regular substitute in a middle–high school until summer, and he had money saved from his island job, so the pressure wasn't great to take just any job. Through the summer and fall, he busied himself with some part-time jobs and doing some building projects around the house for us. But as the time stretched out and no job materialized and his savings ran out, he became more discouraged and somewhat depressed.

As a parent, your feelings move in tandem with your child's, and my wife and I were not immune to this. Two things helped. With Colin, we'd hit walls before, and, working together, we were able to strategize past them, so this gave us some hope. The second was the book. Fortunately for him and for us, he had the book *Smart but Scattered Teens* to work on, and the positive editorial feedback at least stabilized his mood. This also encouraged him to write an article about the potential benefits of some video games for executive skills. With the book done in March, he and his friend got it together, and he did move to Boston in April. He continued to look for work and we helped him with his rent. But by June, he still had no steady work and my wife and I told him, in a phone conversation, that we could not help anymore with rent and he needed to take any job he could find. Within a few weeks he found a job unloading fishing boats at a co-op in New Hampshire, decided that he couldn't afford to stay in Boston full time, and sublet his apartment. Within a month he was a deckhand on a dragger, fishing, which is where he was in the Prologue to this book. For the next 13 months Colin split his time between living with us in New Hampshire and living with his girlfriend in Boston. So after what to us (and perhaps to him, I'm not sure) seemed like a regression, he had landed on his feet and moved on, figuratively and literally, and seemed the stronger and wiser for the experience.

Fast-forward to a year later: Colin moved to St. Louis to be with his girl-friend and started working at a school for children on the moderate-to-severe end of the autism spectrum. It took a while for him to find a job, and during his search he made it clear to my wife and me that he was not going to take just anything that came along. Rather, he wanted to do something that was chal-lenging but also capitalized on some of his previous experience of working with students on the autism spectrum. During the time that he was unemployed our support consisted of health insurance and phone plan payments. He needed occasional other kinds of financial help but for the most part lived off money he had saved from his fishing job and from two royalty checks from his work on *Smart but Scattered Teens.* He did resume an online degree program with con-tinuing ups and downs. We were supporting his education with money from his educational mutual fund that he did not previously use. We also provided some intermittent skill support that we'll have more to say about later in this book. Colin also now had health insurance and retirement fund benefits from his job, along with modest sick leave and vacation time.

Important take-home points about Colin's journey through 2014 include the fact that while he had at times lost steam or even seemed to be going in the wrong direction, the overall trend was toward the goal of independence, and Colin was considerably farther on in that journey than he was a year or two earlier. Another essential fact in this situation was that Colin chose his own direction. A third essential point is that we chose to support him in certain ways that we were comfortable with and that he agreed to.

> Worried that the young adult isn't making any progress toward independence? Look back at the items you checked off on the How Do You Two Define Independence? checklist and ask yourselves if there has been any movement toward accomplishing those goals.

If your young adult is to increase her self-sufficiency and eventually become independent, your assistance and support will be critical. There are three aspects to this support:

1. **Your acceptance of your young adult's goal.** We've touched on the idea that the decision needs to be the young adult's, and we'll get into the practicalities of passing the baton in that way in Step 4.

2. **Your emotional support and words of encouragement and reinforce-ment for her efforts to move forward.** We emphasize the encouragement of effort as opposed to only encouraging goal accomplishment because

the psychological research on motivations indicates that encouraging effort is the most effective way to get individuals to persist in their positive behavior.

3. **Your willingness to offer both skill support and material support.** To accomplish a goal requires a range of skills: for example, planning, time management, focus, and persistence. If your young adult is weak in one or another of these or other associated skills, you may need to provide some support for these skills. Material support might mean assistance with living expenses, rent, health insurance, and finances for training programs or tuition.

To maintain this level of commitment and support of your young adult you need to know that the goal that she has selected is realistic. Does she have the skills and determination to accomplish the goal in what you consider to be a reasonable amount of time? Are her skills well matched or a good fit for the goal that she wants to accomplish? In Step 3 we will provide you with a way to identify the young adult's aptitudes, talents, and skills, so that you can combine this information with the information from Step 1 about her executive skills in identifying realistic goals. For example, if she is more comfortable in a situation with limited social interaction demands, then work involving customer relations or service is not likely to be a good fit. Or, if he struggles with sustaining attention to detail or is impulsive, then air traffic control is probably not a good fit. You get the idea. Goals that are in line with preference and skills have a better chance of being achieved.

These tools will also help you and your young adult understand what specific types of support you can offer to build a bridge to increased self-sufficiency. Once you and your young adult have that information, then you'll be able to determine if the goal is a good fit and therefore reasonable and worthy of your support.

Support as a Collaborator Instead of as a Parent

The fact that your young adult will need your assistance to move ahead creates a tricky balancing act for you. As we've noted, reverting to your traditional parent–child relationship will ensure that the journey to independence remains interrupted. So you need to figuratively move from the driver's seat into the passenger seat, not unlike you literally did when you were working with your child on learning how to drive. If you're going to be effective in this collaborative relationship, you will need to practice restraint.

Let's say your adult child comes up with a proposed plan or goal and you have your doubts about it. Exercising restraint means not criticizing the plan or pointing out why your goals may be more sensible or realistic. We're not suggesting that you unconditionally accept any proposed goal. In a collaborative relationship, your job is to help the young adult gather the information that will let her determine whether what she says she wants to happen can in fact happen. You want her to answer the question of whether there is goodness of fit between her current life situation and skills and the place that she wants to move to next. If her answer is no, you go back to the drawing board to collaborate with her on a new plan that is a good fit as well as a step toward independence. Since in any plan that your young adult proposes she is likely to need ongoing encouragement, emotional support, skills, and probably material support, you will still have a significant decision-making role in the collaboration.

Remember Past Successes

Do you remember the first time your daughter rode off on her bike alone and out of sight? How about leaving her home alone for the first time? Later, watching her drive away in the car on her own for the first time may have been particularly tough. Or when you dropped her off at college or at the airport at the beginning of a trip on her own. The recurring theme here is a period of parental support while children build their skills, followed by taking the risk of letting them go to try these skills independently. In these circumstances we don't typically cut them loose completely, and if they stumble or fall we help them get up, regroup, and try again.

As parents, the stakes for us and for them do get progressively higher because at each new benchmark our children move farther away from us and our protection and guidance. We want them to consider our advice and plan for them to ensure their future security and safety, and thereby alleviate our anxiety. But for the young adult this is meant to be a time of exploration and discovery, a chance to try out a world of new possibilities and an opportunity to find the best fit. Risks and mistakes, as they always have been, are inevitable and necessary for growth and learning to take place. Virtually every young adult has taken risks that, even if they haven't panned out 100%, can be counted as some sort of success. Remembering that independence is a work in progress and that every learning opportunity inches them forward is key.

Also remember that the path to success is not always straight or short. What someone decides to do at 23 or 24 does not doom or restrict the possibilities for her life at 30. Parents often fear that young adults who leave college before graduating, get a job, and get a taste for earning money will never go back to school—a prophecy disproven by the fact that up to 40% of students who leave college return to complete their degrees. Those who do not return cite two primary and related reasons: lack of financial resources and concern about accruing more debt and the stress of balancing school and work in order to avoid greater debt. My own experience suggests a third reason. Both of our children dropped out of college. Neither showed an inclination to return or the motivation to succeed until they had each identified a career goal (behavior analyst, nurse) that demanded a degree. In addition, as we discuss elsewhere in this book, college is not the only path to success by a long shot.

Acceptance, Emotional Support, and Moral Support

In our work with young adults who are not moving forward, one of the recurring roadblocks to change involves discouragement and lack of confidence. These feelings of young adults arise, among other causes, out of a sense of failing to meet adult expectations—those of parents, teachers, job supervisors. As a parent you can positively affect your young adult's self-confidence. In fact, you've already taken a significant step in this direction if you've agreed to collaborate with the young adult on a particular goal. In addition, although it might not seem like much, simply making yourself available to listen to your young adult's ideas without criticizing them can have great benefits. For young adults, talking about ideas and hopes is a way to test the water of what's out in the world without major risk or effort and is also a way to test out parental support and reaction.

In *Motivational Interviewing with Adolescents and Young Adults*, authors Naar-King and Suarez discuss "change talk," noting that it is critical to maintain a nonjudgmental attitude toward young adults regardless of what we think may be the unrealistic nature of their ideas, since the end result is still their increased motivation for change. In moving into this collaborative relationship and supporting your young adult to more independently negotiate the real world, you are taking yourself out of the "expert" or "I know best" role that you've played through much of your child's development and instead pointing him toward "real world" experts (bankers, doctors, mechanics, lawyers) to help guide him. Simply by doing this you've facilitated his transition to the real world and given the young adult an opportunity to practice a skill that needs to be practiced and internalized. The following dialogues characterize two different stances that a parent can take, the first undermining and the second facilitating independence.

"Is there any more milk?"

"Well, you're looking in the right place."

"I know. Is there any more though?"

"Cass, you're looking in the only place." Keith stopped putting rinsed dishes on a towel next to the sink and looked over at his 23-year-old daughter.

"Listen, Dad, I gotta tell you something." Abrupt segues were the norm for Cassandra. Keith was used to them by now, though he made it known that for his money, phones were to blame; he called it text-message-locution-mission-creep.

"What, Cass?" he said with mock import.

"I'm thinking about moving down to Ridley, you know, closer to the city. I thought maybe it'd let me check out what's downtown easier, for jobs and stuff."

Keith's light tone faded quickly. "So to recap, you've just decided that you are maybe moving to Ridley, because maybe it will be easier there to maybe find a job, or 'stuff,' downtown?"

"Well, no, I mean I've thought about it a lot, I talked to Kate, and she said that things are goo-"

"Kate lives in Ridley, doesn't she?"

"Well, yeah and—"

"No."

"No?"

"No."

"No what, Dad?"

"No whatever, Cass. No, I don't think it's a good idea. No, I don't like it. No, I won't support it. No, I don't really trust you living with Kate, or really Kate's judgment in general. So take your pick, no." Keith's rising inflection at the end of each statement made him sound like a Valley girl, but Cass wasn't in the mood.

"Whoa, let's back up a second, Dad. First, I don't know why your opinion of Kate—wrong by the way—is relevant here, but thanks for that. Second, I'm not walking into this blind. A lot of people my age are down there for good reasons; yes because 'there are bars there that aren't also diners' as you've said before, but the area is safe and affordable, and look at the job market in the city! If I'm looking for experience in marketing and sales, then it makes all the sense in the world to go there."

"Affordable. Affordable? Affordable for who? Do you have a job downtown? Is Kate going to pay your rent? Affordability is determined by *whoever is paying, and barring any employment revelation you're about to share, I think that whoever is your mom and I."*

"What are you talking about? I don't know how we got here, but in case you've forgotten, I'm paying to be here now! I'm paying to be here now because you and Mom thought it would make me want to get my own place, and congratulations—it worked! So what, Dad? I'm s'posed to grab my crystal ball and tell you down to the friggin' fine print how this is going to work? It's like you just want to tell me I'm wrong, just for the self-satisfaction of looking like the wiser person."

"You really think that's my agenda here? You said so yourself; we want you to move out and be on your own! But we aren't going to subsidize some indefinite sabbatical in Ridley while you casually discover your path!"

"So then the alternative is no path?!"

"Cass, we're doing dinner soon," Keith said, rubbing his forehead, "I just don't—can't do this right now."

"And I hadn't planned to do this either. You brought us here. But whatever, I'll grab something to eat later."

Alternate Ending

"No."

"No?"

"No."

Cassandra sighed, grabbed a soda from the fridge, and smiled slightly as she picked up a clean glass from the towel and looked at her father.

"Wow, Dad, this glass is super clean."

Keith looked at her with reserved surprise and said with mock sarcasm, "Why, thank you, dear! I credit my special drying technique, which I honed when—"

"When you washed dishes at that diner in Pittsburgh? I know, Dad, you've told me, several times, and several more times after that. In fact you lived above that diner, didn't you? Because it was the only job you could find that let you live in the city and finish night school?"

Keith wagged his finger in the air, "Walked uphill both ways in the snow! With no 4G coverage!"

"And didn't you do that because you were trying to get a job at a bank when you finished?"

"Yes! And I got the job and hated it and moved back into the hill country!"

"Hill country? Simmer down, Dad. You moved like 30 minutes from Pittsburgh, not exactly 'Into the Wild.' And I get your point, it didn't work out for you. But you gave it a shot, and came out of it okay, and you always reference it as an important time in your life."

Keith looked over at his daughter and let out a deep breath, "Yeah, yeah, okay, I finished night school, so I know where you're going with this. But listen, things didn't completely fall apart for me and the experience taught me a lot, but that doesn't mean it was easy or that I don't regret any part of it. I was broke, alone, and stressed out for a long time while I was there. It worked out, but it could have gone better, and when I look at you outlining this plan it sounds all too familiar, and I don't want you to go through what I did when you don't have to."

"I can understand that, Dad. But what if it does work out for me? I know you see all these parallels, but your life isn't like cheat codes for mine."

"No, but it should inform yours. And the finance, the money issue? That's real, this isn't living with us, it's signing leases and paying bills and paying parking tickets and checking the mail every day and . . . and washing the dishes!"

"Then help me learn them, Dad. I see what you're saying, but that means it's a catch-22 for me; stay here because I don't do those things, don't do those things when I stay here."

Keith nodded. "Dinner's soon. Okay, Cass, that's a valid argument. After we eat, if you want to sit down, we'll go over what a hypothetical apartment would look like and how it would operate, and maybe get some budget ideas on paper. Deal?"

Cassandra smiled, "Deal."

"Good. Now, in the meantime, see how I rotate the bottom of the glass, using minimal finger contact, while wiping in concentric circles around the rim area with the dish towel? It's about speed, about touch, you want to wipe firmly, but avoid a hard scrubbing motion, it'll leave visible fibers. See Cass? Cass?" Keith glanced up and saw her looking at her phone.

"Text-message-locution-creep! It's an epidemic!" he cried.

"Calm down, Dad. I'm looking at dishwashers."

In this second dialogue, Keith is taking himself out of the "parent" (hierarchical) decision-making role and instead accepting the young adult's plan. He's working collaboratively with her to give her the best chance of success while at the same time finding an opportunity to use his experience and mitigate some of the risks.

Don't mistake "staying out of it" for acceptance. Stepping aside, ostensibly so the young adult can take his "best shot," can masquerade as respecting the young adult's autonomy. If you've decided that staying silent and not erecting roadblocks is a way to give your child the freedom to decide for himself, take a moment to examine your reasons and make sure your goal is sincerely to give the young adult a chance at decision making. Sometimes we tell ourselves if the child fails he'll see the advantage or superiority of our plan over his—an agenda that is more common the wider the gap between what we believe is the right course and what the young adult believes is best for him. This scenario can make it pretty difficult to resist the "I told you so" urge. The only time when stepping aside in passive "support" makes sense is when the young adult explicitly states, "I want to try this on my own and I'll come to you when/if I need help," *and* you believe the young adult's plan has a realistic chance of success. Then, if agreed-upon benchmarks and timelines (discussed in later steps) are not met, and the young adult doesn't approach you for help, you'll need to make the first move and engage in collaborative problem solving rather than remaining passive and waiting for a recovery that may not come.

Emotional support means encouraging the young adult's efforts and accepting her autonomy and decision making, including listening as a sounding board, while refraining from correction or criticism. For example, "It sounds like you've got a starting point that you're comfortable with, and it's worked well for you in the past. Try it out if you're ready, let me know how it's going, and tell me if there's anything I can do to help."

Skill Support and Material/Financial Support

Another type of support your adult child might need is help to develop or strengthen a skill if he is not sure how to proceed. For example, the young adult may have a reasonable goal but be unsure of the specific steps to get the process started or keep it moving along due to lack of planning skills and experience. In this case, you want to help with the planning process through a series of questions and discussions involving different options, *without* prescribing your own plan in detail, which would only undermine the young adult's autonomy and put you back in the parent or expert role.

Another type of support might come in the form of financial assistance. For example, if your daughter says, "I think my chances for getting this job would be good if I got this training certificate. Can you help me pay for it?," you need to know whether that job is a goal she has examined for goodness of fit, whether you think her assessment seems realistic, whether she has the executive skills to successfully complete the training, and under what conditions you're willing to offer this financial support. In fact, it's critical before agreeing to provide material or financial support that you know fully and realistically what you're getting into so you can ensure that you're prepared to stick out any agreement you arrive at.

What kind of tangible supports are you willing to invest?

- College tuition or other educational fees? How much, where, and for what degree or certificate? Are there any conditions for your paying for school?

- A place to live? At home with you or somewhere else? For free or with a partial rent contribution from you?

- A car or other transportation assistance to get to school or a job?

> Be sure you know fully what you're getting into before committing to support so you can follow through on the agreement.

Obviously you'll have to make more specific, concrete decisions on support once a goal is selected and you and the young adult know what kinds of assistance reaching it will require, but it's good to start thinking about what you're prepared to do.

How Much Support Is Too Much?

This is a tough question to answer, because it's so individual. But if your young adult has a comfortable lifestyle and envisions that what is to be gained by increased self-sufficiency and independence is a decline in lifestyle, why would she strive for independence? If you think this might be the case, you may have to consider making what are currently the young adult's preferences and comforts available only if she makes some concrete contribution to the household in terms of chores or finances. They might include, for example, access to a computer and the Internet, cable television programs, money or transportation for entertainment, and so forth. For parents who are either not used to or out of practice with limit setting for their children, this can be difficult. If you're not sure what to do or are uncomfortable imposing these limits but understand the need, we recommend seeking out the help of a coach or more likely a counselor who can serve as a negotiator. (See Step 9.)

The Fading of the "American Dream"

Unfortunately, there's another factor today that can have an impact on how much support may feel like too much. There is a general consensus that the

"American Dream" of going to college, getting a well-paying job, and achieving financial stability and comfort is harder to achieve than we thought and that we may have led our children to believe. For example, some college graduates are taking lower-skilled jobs that don't require bachelor's degrees, and this comes at a time when "middle-class" jobs such as teaching, sales agents, and financial analysts are shrinking. Young adults also are holding fewer full-time jobs than in previous years. A Federal Reserve study published at the end of 2016 indicated that nearly half of college graduates are underemployed and working jobs that don't require BAs. In addition, the likelihood that young adults will earn more than their parents has fallen in dramatic fashion within the last few decades. Of young adults born in 1984, just half earned more than their parents at age 30.

As a parent, what are you to do in this situation? On the one hand, you can feel understandable empathy for your young adult's plight and acknowledge that it's based on economic factors that she may not be able to control. On the other hand, if discouragement and fear of failure have already derailed her, your continuing support threatens to solidify this stance. This is even more likely when the young adult's lifestyle at home is better than she is likely to achieve quickly on her own. At the same time, you both recognize (hopefully) that this situation cannot continue indefinitely, so you need to find ways to enhance the young adult's readiness to change.

Is the Young Adult Ready (Motivated) to Change?

If the young adult is to move forward toward independence, his or her readiness for change is essential. On what does readiness for change depend? In a word, *motivation*—readiness for change is basically a measure of a person's motivational state. When a person says she is ready to change, that means that she is at the starting line and committed to putting forward the effort to get to the finish line. What is it that motivates a young adult and readies her to invest effort into change? A goal—but it can't be just any goal. According to the psychological research on goals, the young adult must be enthused about the goal and believe that she can actually achieve it.

But how does she really know? Perhaps she believes she has the aptitude or skills to achieve the goal. Or, if she is not quite there with the skills, maybe she believes she has the aptitude and will have the support to get the skills she needs. In other words, she has reason to be confident. But is this confidence built on solid evidence? Since parents are part of this equation, it's fair for you to ask if this confidence is supported by the facts.

Or maybe the problem is that even readiness for change is weak or absent due to insufficient motivation. Young adults who have experienced a failure or series of failures in meeting their goals are likely to be discouraged or depressed. Depending on where the young adult falls on the continuum of these emotions, going through the assessment and planning process described in the following steps, along with parental encouragement and assurances of

> *If the road to hell can be paved with good intentions, it can also be paved with false confidence.*

support, may be enough to get him started and moving ahead. *But if you suspect your young adult is depressed or he or she acknowledges depression, it's important to address the depression with a professional.* Even minor setbacks in the change process can, for a depressed young adult, exacerbate feelings of depression. See Step 9.

Lack of Confidence

What else drains motivation? Maybe your young adult is not quite sure of a direction to move in, as is the case for Jonas; he lacks a goal or at least a goal that's obvious at the moment. Or, perhaps the young adult does have a goal but either doesn't know how to get there or doubts, in his heart of hearts, that he can get there. If one or more past experiences of not achieving a goal has led him to anticipate failure, maybe he's reluctant to risk another failure. He could have confidence in the goal but not in the support needed to reach it. This might be the case if he did not have the financial resources needed to return to school or to relocate for a job prospect.

Parental Coercion

Then there are the parent factors. Parents also play a significant role in readiness for change and motivation. Cassandra was motivated by her readiness to move to the city with her friend. Her dad's initial rejection of this plan stopped Cass in her tracks, but he was able to get on board to at least reconsider this opportunity for her. Chris's mother, on the other hand, erected a subtle roadblock to Chris's persistence and even hinted at retribution:

> *"Hi, Mom, how's it going?"*
> *"Hey Chris, good, good. How are you?"*
> *"Oh you know just the usual. Work, watching TV now. Where are you?"*

"Well, I'm leaving work soon and heading to get your sister from basketball practice."

"Oh, cool."

"Anyway, the reason I'm calling is that I saw Carl's dad, Mark or Marcus I think his name is, at Dunkin' Donuts earlier."

"Oh yeah? How's shmfggfsin . . . sorry, I'm eating pretzels. How's he doing? Carl I mean."

"Oh he's good! Mark said Carl just passed his Series Six exam [to become an investment company products representative], so he'll be putting in for a transfer to a larger branch at LifeCo."

"Oh, awesome! That's cool."

"Yeah. So anyway, Carl said LifeCo was going to pay for Carl's MBA. Didn't you guys have the same major at PFU?"

"Yeah, well, Carl had a different focus, but yeah, we both did communications."

"Right. Well, maybe you should consider that. I know of a few places around here that are looking for tellers or salespeople; you should see if they would offer the same thing."

"Hahaha. Mom, my concentration was more on mass media and stuff. I don't want to be a bank teller, I want to work at a tech place or start-up. I don't know if I could even get into an MBA program."

"Well, yes, I know you say that, but just look at Carl. He's got stability—they're paying for him to go back to school to get a better job. What's better than that?"

"Mom, that's great for Carl. I have zero interest in finance. I've always been good with computers, I get this stuff, this is what I want to do. Jimkam isn't Facebook, but I'm getting experience."

"A couple computers in a closet-sized office just isn't a business, Chris. The whole reason I am where I am is that I stayed at Liberty and took the sure thing. I want to see you succeed, that's all. What if I paid for your MBA? Call it an interest-free loan. You can do all sorts of things with it, even work at a tech company!"

"Yeah, I don't want an MBA, though, Mom. I'm not fascinated by that stuff. I'm not any good at it either. I appreciate it, though. What if I could go back for an associate's degree or certificate in coding? I know a lot already. It would give me the flexibility to take a variety of positions at the types of places I find appealing."

"Well, you can ask your father. But it just doesn't seem like a sound investment to me. If you know it already, then just learn it in your free *time. Coding? No one cares about your degree; they just want you to know how to write code. But the MBA is a ticket you can cash anywhere—it has value."*

"Not true, Mom, but whatever. Listen, I appreciate your offer, but I like what I'm doing. I just can't see myself being in that field, so I'll keep going at Jimkam and continue to look for other options."

"Well, okay, sweetie, it's your life. Speaking of which, though, we do need to talk about our kind of medium- to long-term ideas about your living arrangements. I think it's probably fair that you should pay some sort of rent if Jimkam is what you think you're going to be doing for the foreseeable future."

"Um, jeez. Okay, well, you know I'm not exactly making tons of money, so I'm not sure how much I can afford, but yeah, if you want to talk about it that's cool. I guess I'll see you when I get home."

"Okay. I'm going to get your sister now. If there's something you need, just text me."

"Okay, thanks. Hey, Mom, this rent thing, is this about the MBA thing?"

"Oh, no, Chris. I've been thinking about it for a little while now. I just feel that you maybe need to figure out how to manage things when you're on a budget. And I could always use the extra cash for things around the house . . ."

"Oh, okay then. Well, see you soon, Mom."

"Okay, Chris, bye."

Even though in this circumstance Chris's mother feels that she has her son's best interest at heart and wants only what she believes is best for him, she is unfortunately directly undermining his autonomy by attempting to coerce him to do what she wants him to do. Coercion like this is likely to fail. The agenda may already have failed in the past, in that the young adult likely signed on to a parent goal (e.g., a degree, a certain professional track or career) and couldn't achieve that goal, which is how he ended in this current position. Coercion for the young adult can easily hark back to late adolescence, when he may have more actively rejected your bidding as a way to establish his own decision making and autonomy.

When the young adult's chosen goal seems realistic and meets our criteria for furthering independence, it deserves parental support. But if you feel the young adult's goal is shortsighted or offers no opportunity for advancement, or it doesn't reach the level of achievement or status that you feel is important for your young adult's future or your self-esteem, you may be tempted to try to coerce the young adult to see things your way. If your young adult listens to your opinion but rejects it and you're okay with this, you've sidestepped the temptation to coerce. But if you actively or passively withhold emotional, skill, and/or material support, or if you attempt to leverage the support so that it is contingent on the young adult's adopting in part or in whole what you believe is a better goal, you're heading down a path that not only leads away from independence but can also create resentment.

Moving Forward

Regarding adult children living with parents, an article posted by the Clay Center for Healthy Young Minds at Massachusetts General Hospital indicated that in this situation young adults are susceptible to increased psychological distress, strained peer relations due to lack of privacy, and a sense of regression to an earlier stage of development. For both parents and young adults, this results in role confusion, ambivalence about their relationship, and uncertainty about what the future holds.

To combat these potential issues, we recommend the following:

- Have a written plan, a timeline, and specific steps and measures that indicate that the young adult is becoming more self-sufficient.

- Offer material support as a help, not a handout. Money is preferably for activities that foster independence, such as for gas for work. If the amount of money is significant and involves education or training, have the young adult take out loans that you will cosign for.

- Support to get to the destination should be modest. A rowboat or skiff, not a super yacht; food, clothing, shelter, health insurance, car (maybe); and perhaps a phone. Frequent meals out, bar hopping, and high-end vacations are not part of the package.

- Help the young adult build financial and work habits (we'll get specific in Step 9). If he can't currently contribute financially, have him contribute in kind through chores and jobs around the house, such as babysitting/ ride for siblings or cleaning. Work with him to prepare a budget so he will understand day-to-day living expenses for what he will need when he moves out.

Note that education and/or training are generally worthy of parental support with these cautions: Does the proposed education or training move the young adult toward an identifiable job or career? What performance criteria and timelines need to be met for continued support? In the case of education or training, having the young adult take out loans to support her goals in part meets the criteria for "skin in the game." Depending on where the young adult is in the process, you might also want to consider financial support for some type of career or vocational assessment since this may yield directional information.

> *Whenever considering support, ask yourself, "Are the money and resources I am providing fostering independence or extending dependence?"*

In this step, we've tried to get you and your young adult thinking about how ready you both are to move forward:

- How ready is the young adult to start moving away from total dependence on you and toward some form of independence? How motivated is he to keep at it? Is he pretty happy where he is or eager to get out and get going?

- Have you been able to agree on what independence means at this point? Does it mean the young adult's taking on more responsibilities at the house, more personal care, contributing to the household like another adult living there, or making bigger leaps, like moving out with a job that will pay the rent?

- Does the young adult have a goal of some kind, or is she completely stymied, unable to budge out of childhood behavior and attitudes, unprepared to make any decisions about moving forward?

- Can you two capitalize on what has worked for you in the past when your child needed to make some step toward greater independence to start a productive collaboration?

- Can you shift toward being an active collaborator and supporter and away from calling the shots?

- Are you ready and willing to help your child make his own decisions about his future and to help him fulfill his dreams even if they are not your dreams for him?

There's no denying that when young adults are at a standstill it's almost always the result of factors involving the child *and* the parent. Is the young adult really as unmotivated as you believe? Or are you sending mixed messages? Expecting adult behavior but treating the young adult like a child? Telling the young adult he has to "stand on his own two feet" but then making living at home way too comfortable for him to leave? The dynamics between you and your adult child have been carved out in your relationship over years, and they aren't always easy to bring into sharp relief or to change, so we've devoted an entire chapter (Step 4) to what you, individually, can do to hand off the baton, respect boundaries, and allow your child to claim the independence you say you want her to achieve. If you want to help your adult child succeed, you need to ensure there's a good fit between you two in this collaboration. But now let's shift the focus to your young adult. Young adults who are stalled often have trouble establishing and meeting a specific goal toward independence because they really don't know themselves very well. In the next step they have the opportunity to step back and get to know themselves and what type of adult life might be a good fit for them.

STEP 3

· ·

Identify a Realistic Direction
The Young Adult's Interests and Aptitudes

When we left them in Chapter 2, Jonas's mother, Marta, had just reiterated a point she feels like she's made a thousand times over the last few years since he dropped out of college: she wanted him to "start again" to try to figure out what he wants to do with his life.

> *"I know, I know," her son replies. "Well, and I want to too. I want to get on track and do something and move out. And I know what you mean: sometimes it feels like I'm too well adjusted, like I go to work and come back and forget that I want something else for myself. But I dunno, a lot of stuff that I think about ends up like the IT thing. Like I think about it, or I'm interested in the idea of it, but when I try to imagine what it might be like to work a job like that, I just can't envision it. And that makes me think it's not for me. All my friends and stuff talk about passion or that they're really into their jobs, or that at least they're sticking it out for the money or the opportunity. I feel like I've never had anything that grabbed me that way. I feel like I semi-enjoy a lot of things, but there's not anything I know about that I love or feel like 'Aha, now that's what I should be.' "*
>
> *"Well, first of all I don't think that that way of thinking is as rare as maybe your perception makes it out to be," Marta replies. "Some people aren't passionate about their jobs, others become passionate about their jobs while they're employed, others just convince themselves that they are really invigorated by what they do but they aren't. But—and trust me, Jonas, I'm not trying to be that mom—but have you taken any questionnaires or tests*

to see what you might like? Or not even what you like, but what type of job you might be good at?"

"I mean maybe, like in high school I think we took some surveys along those lines. But otherwise no, not really. I have a hard time buying into that idea that a test will just tell me what I should do."

"True, and I don't think it will tell you what your ideal job is. But I think you should try some of these. Not as a definitive answer on who you are and what you should do, but just use them, use them as a tool to help you think about things. Not an exact job but just more types of work. Because I think in any area there are all different kinds of jobs that suit different people. So being good at math doesn't mean you have to be an engineer or an accountant, and being introverted doesn't mean you should get a job that never requires you to interact with people. But just take a look at these. Even if you don't fill out the answers right away, at least think about some of the questions. Or take them 10 different times and see if and how your answers change. I don't think they're supposed to tell you what to do. They're just supposed to help you tell yourself what to do. That make sense? Or am I just being too vague and talking in circles?"

"Well, you are, but that's nothing new." Jonas cracked a small grin at his mother's mock offense. "I get it, though, what you're getting at. Don't take the questionnaires literally as gospel; treat them more like a prompt or something."

"Exactly."

The questionnaires Marta is recommending to Jonas include the Executive Skills Questionnaire you've already seen in Step 1 and one presented in this chapter that's designed to help young adults figure out what their preferences and aptitudes are and what talents and skills they have that might factor into making a living and finding a direction toward independence.

Goodness of Fit

In Step 1 we noted that to move forward young adults need to define a goal that is a good fit with their executive skills. In assessing your young adult's executive skills strengths and weaknesses you two gained a new lens through which to view what's holding the young adult back. Are his executive skills underdeveloped to the point of paralysis? Young men and women who can't initiate, plan, or follow through due to a number of executive skills weaknesses may have a lot of trouble even envisioning becoming self-sufficient, much less getting to the launching pad. Other young adults have tried living on their own, pursuing higher education, or dabbled in various occupations, only to bounce back home with depleted financial and emotional resources. Their executive skills profile can reveal a lot about why these efforts may have been doomed from the outset.

Or maybe not. Their disappointments might have resulted instead from discovering that the chosen direction left them as uninspired and unmotivated as Jonas fears he will be in IT or Chris knew he would be in finance. The factors discussed in Step 2 can leave a young adult unmotivated or unready for change, but the motivation gap can also emerge when the young adult doesn't know himself well enough to identify a road worth following.

Gina figured she was a natural to follow in her RN (registered nurse) mom's footsteps. At her daycare job, she was the go-to person for bruised knees and runny noses. True, she had a hiccup with chem in high school, but her counselor figured with her motivation she'd manage, yet by the end of first semester, discouraged, she bailed on school and her RN dream.

> *When a bump in the road flattens your tire or a roadblock requires a detour, how do you resist the urge to turn back if the destination (or the joy of the ride) isn't that compelling?*

Dion grew up doing 4-H club, so animal care was in his blood. Veterinarian seemed like the perfect choice. After a year of tough courses and a meeting with his advisor, he realized he was looking at seven or more additional years of this grind to hit his goal. He had imagined himself as a vet but not the road to get there. Discouraged, he withdrew to rethink his career choice.

English lit degree in hand, Jayden thought he was home-free. College grads were more employable and earned more money, right? He loved the writing and analysis in English lit, but he had no interest in teaching and couldn't see how his interest translated into a job that was stimulating and gave him enough to live on.

Goal setting by the young adult and your support of your son or daughter's goal is the necessary foundation for the young adult's journey to independence, because having a goal motivates and energizes us. We're willing to make sacrifices and learn skills if they will help us get to our goal, and we'll persist as long as the goal is in sight and we think we can reach it. This is as true for young adults as it is for parents.

When roadblocks halt the young adult's progress, both of you might start to feel uncertain about the direction the young adult has chosen or doubtful about the chance of success. To get past these doubts you both need some assurance that the young adult has chosen a path and a goal that can be achieved because it's a good fit with the adult's abilities. For the young adult who is stuck and perhaps frustrated or discouraged, having confidence in her ability to succeed as well as experiencing initial success is key to maintaining momentum and building independence.

You've already looked at one of the two major components essential to achieving a chosen goal: goodness of fit between the goal and the young adult's executive skills profile (Step 1). The second, covered in this chapter, is goodness of fit between the young adult's skills and preferences and the chosen goal. Here we are talking about academic and work skills that have been acquired through school, training, or work experience. Preferences include free-time pursuits, social activities, desired living and work environments, and school preferences if the young adult is considering a return to school.

Gina's goal didn't fit because her executive skills weakness in sustaining attention came into play when her interest in a course was low and effort was high. Her interest in health care and biology classes wasn't enough to carry her through less-appealing requirements. After talking with her mom, she realized it wasn't runny noses but working with little kids that appealed to her, and she moved into early childhood studies. Goal-directed persistence was a relative strength for Dion as long as the goal was within his time horizon. Seven or more years before he could practice was not. But a co-op college program in veterinary technology gave him an immediate chance to do what he loved, hands-on work with animals in an internship, and a 3-year completion date, which was a great fit. Jayden knew he had interest in English and writing, but since teaching was out, he couldn't see options that appealed and could give him enough to live on. A friend of his working at a biotech company said they were interviewing for technical writers. It didn't sound appealing, but he needed a job. The interviewer, himself an English major, hit it off with Jayden, and he landed the job. It turned out that he had a knack for translating complex information into understandable English, and he found he enjoyed the challenge.

Goal selection could begin with fantasizing about what the young adult might want to do in life—there's nothing wrong with brainstorming and using the power of imagination. But fantasy doesn't spell success. Successful goal selection begins instead by matching up a dream goal with the reality of who the young adult is, what she likes, what academic or work skills she has, and what skills she needs to learn to be successful. A goal based on this information will set the stage for building

> *To be realistically achievable, a goal needs to match a dream with the reality of who the young adult is.*

a plan. It will help young adults and parents identify the tools needed to construct a road map to the goal as well as the potential obstacles. This information, in turn, will help parents know what supports will be necessary to bypass roadblocks, feel confident that the goal is realistic, and be willing to provide support.

The Getting to Know Myself Questionnaire

In this chapter we offer a questionnaire that we've developed as a tool for the young adult to spell out his or her talents, likes and dislikes, skills and experiences. The Getting to Know Myself Questionnaire (GTKMQ) is based on our clinical work with emerging adults. We have worked in coaching sessions with these young adults and their parents to help the young adults sort out their priorities and provide sufficient information to discuss goals or potential goals. Young adults using this questionnaire have told us that spelling out their skills and preferences has given them a direction for their efforts. It is modeled on a questionnaire we published in our book *The Smart but Scattered Guide to Success* (see the Resources for details).

The objective is for the young adult and parents to examine the results and, with a particular emphasis on interests, talents, and skills, discuss what direction this information points to. In some cases, the information will serve to confirm a goal that the young adult has considered and establish the beginnings of a road map for how to get there. Jonas's questionnaire results point in this direction. In other cases, the results will offer a jumping-off point for brainstorming possible trajectories when the young adult has no goal in mind.

A few tips to keep in mind before you begin:

1. *If using the questionnaire is your idea (vs. the young adult's, if he's reading this book), present it as just a prompt*—something to get the young adult thinking and the two of you talking constructively. If the young adult has felt cajoled or coerced into pursuing a goal he wasn't sure of and he hasn't gotten anywhere, he may hesitate to take any step that might lead him to a conclusion he'll feel stuck with. Take a page from Marta.

2. *Be prepared to be open to whatever results emerge.* Look at the results for points of emphasis or a recurring theme and use it as a catalyst for conversation. Resist any urge to interpret the results as an indication that your preferred goal is where goodness of fit lies for your young adult.

3. *Be sure to convey that you'll hear out whatever ideas the questionnaire stimulates in your young adult.* Remember that this may be the young adult's first concrete step toward identifying or clarifying a goal that will motivate him. Young adults need to feel free to offer their information and opinions, without comments, limitations, or critical feedback. You are not signing on to their goals at this point, so you need not question or critique what the young adult chooses to respond with. Your opportunity to ask questions about how "realistic" the goal that is ultimately chosen is will come after the information-gathering part of this process is complete. While it may not seem like a big deal, keep this point in mind. There are risks in this process for both you and the young adult. How your collaborative efforts as a parent can help the two of you avoid them is addressed in Step 4.

Young adults can fill in the questionnaire on pages 72–75, but it's also available online for those who want to fill it in more than once (interests and preferences can certainly change over time); see the end of the Contents for information.

Looking at the Getting to Know Myself Questionnaire Results

Unless they're involved in some sort of formal vocational or career evaluation, most young adults and their parents don't engage in this process of identifying skills and interests in concrete terms. It's our experience that the questionnaire can help both young adults and their parents discover previously unrecognized skills and interests, and these discoveries stimulate thought and discussion and start pointing to a direction for the goal selection process.

Privately reviewing questionnaire results before talking about them with your young adult can head off any impulsive negative response to what you learn.

If you're already amicably working through this book together, the young adult will probably be willing to share the results with you. If not, she may at least be willing to tell you what insights she has gained, and once you gain some ideas for strengthening collaboration in Step 4, she may end up willing to share the actual filled-out questionnaire.

If your young adult allows, look at her responses alone or with your spouse first. This private review allows you time to process the information and inhibit any impulsive emotional responses you might have to information that is disappointing or unexpected.

Getting to Know Myself Questionnaire

Name: _____ Date: _____

1. How do you spend your spare time? Check (✓) all that apply and draw a circle around your favorite three activities.

   Do you prefer to spend free time primarily:

   Social

   - ☐ with family
   - ☐ with friends
   - ☐ with friends on social media
   - ☐ alone
   - ☐ other: _____

   Watching/thinking

   - ☐ playing video games
   - ☐ watching TV/DVDs
   - ☐ using computer (e.g., web surfing, YouTube videos)
   - ☐ listening to music
   - ☐ reading
   - ☐ writing
   - ☐ other: _____

   Hands on

   - ☐ doing arts/crafts
   - ☐ building things
   - ☐ making videos
   - ☐ dirt-biking/four-wheeling
   - ☐ hiking/walking
   - ☐ traveling
   - ☐ sports
   - ☐ working out
   - ☐ playing an instrument
   - ☐ theater/dance
   - ☐ volunteering
   - ☐ other: _____

2. What talents do you have? Check all that apply and provide an example if you can.

   - ☐ athletic: _____
   - ☐ musical: _____
   - ☐ visual arts: _____
   - ☐ performing arts: _____
   - ☐ mechanical skills: _____
   - ☐ cooking: _____
   - ☐ other: _____
   - ☐ sewing: _____
   - ☐ writing: _____
   - ☐ leadership: _____
   - ☐ technology: _____
   - ☐ math/sciences: _____
   - ☐ interpersonal skills: _____

(continued)

3. What personal qualities do you have that you consider to be strengths? Check up to five.

☐ leadership	☐ patience	☐ creativity	☐ sense of humor
☐ independence	☐ caring, empathy	☐ hard worker	☐ loyalty
☐ imagination	☐ dependability	☐ determination	☐ optimism
☐ self-control	☐ coping skills	☐ problem solving	☐ persistence
☐ ambition	☐ honesty	☐ organization	☐ courage
☐ competitiveness	☐ extraversion (outgoing)	☐ working well with others	☐ other: _____ _____

4. What life experiences have you had that you loved, that meant a lot to you, or that you felt you got a lot out of?

_____

_____

_____

_____

5. What areas of skill or knowledge would you like to become an expert in? List *any* topic that interests you, even if it is something you don't usually learn about in school (e.g., video games, sports statistics, fashion design, car repair).

_____

_____

_____

_____

6. What are your educational experiences? Check those that apply.

☐ did not finish high school

☐ high school diploma or ged

☐ high school vocational/technical certification

☐ if no degree, # of credits: _____

☐ college

☐ associate's degree: major: _____

☐ bachelor's degree: major: _____

☐ other training or certificates: _____ _____

(continued)

7. What were your best subjects in school? _____

   And your worst? _____

8. What work experiences have you had? Check all that apply and, on the lines provided, specify the type of job and estimate the number of hours worked per week.

   _____ Part-time

   Jobs: # hours worked per week

   _____

   _____

   _____

   _____ Full-time

   Jobs: # hours worked per week

   _____

   _____

   _____

   _____ Volunteer/internships

   Jobs: # hours worked per week

   _____

   _____

   _____

9. What jobs did you like most? _____

   _____

   _____

10. What jobs did you like least? _____

    _____

    _____

(continued)

11. If you have a choice, where would you prefer to live?

    City, suburb, rural area, etc.: _____

    Which area of the United States (East Coast, Midwest, West Coast, North, South, etc.), or other country? _____

12. What type of job would you like to be working at in 2 years' time? _____

    _____

    What type of job would you like to be working at in 6–8 years' time? _____

    _____

13. If you are currently working, over the next 12–18 months do you intend to:

    ☐ Stay in your current job   ☐ Look for a different job

    ☐ Start or return to school   ☐ Start a training program

    ☐ Not sure

14. If you intend to return to school or a training program, what would you like to study or what skills do you want to learn? _____

    _____

15. What type of school would you prefer?

    ☐ vocational/technical school   ☐ 2-year community college

    ☐ 4-year liberal arts college   ☐ 2–4-year science/technology school

    ☐ 2–4-year business school   ☐ 2–4-year health sciences (e.g., nursing, medical technology) school

    ☐ graduate/professional school

16. Who is going to pay for school?

    ☐ I am, with savings and/or financial aid

    ☐ I am, with loans and financial aid

    ☐ My parents and I together

    ☐ My parents

Possible Conversation Starters

Once you've looked at the responses and had a chance to process the information, the following are possible questions for launching further discussions:

- "Derek, when we've talked before, it sounded like you were interested in _____. After doing the questionnaire, what direction do you see yourself maybe moving in? What are you seeing as some ways to get there or move in that direction?"

- "I know you said before, Justine, that you didn't know what would appeal to you or suit you. In thinking about this information now, what might appeal to you? Not necessarily a job or career, I mean, but maybe where you'd like to live or the kind of people you'd like to work with?"

- "ML, I feel like I learned some things about you I didn't know, like your interest in _____. Tell me more about it; I'd love to know."

- (For the young adult who already has a goal in mind that you two are discussing) "JT, it sounds like your responses pretty much confirm what you were already planning for. If you're going to move ahead, what other questions or concerns do you need to manage? Or are there any potential roadblocks? If so, how are you thinking about getting past them?"

The first three questions are open ended for a reason: to get to whatever your young adult is thinking, without imposing your own expectations. The last question is multifaceted and gets at subjects that we'll explore more fully in later steps, but don't miss the opportunity to see what new issues the questionnaire brings up even when it confirms the overall proposed goal.

KEY POINTS TO REMEMBER ABOUT THE GTKMQ

- This is an information exchange.
- Ask open-ended questions.
- Be as neutral as possible. This is not a one-time, do-or-die conversation.

What the Questionnaire Can Reveal

- Some of the reasons young adults make the choices they make
- Why some situations are more likely than others to be successful for them

- Why *parents'* earlier goals for the young adult may not have been successful
- What direction the young adult wants to move in
- Types of directions that do not make sense because they are a poor fit with who the young adult is
- An idea of the kinds of supports the young adult might need to reach that future goal

If Dion had filled out the questionnaire before choosing his college major, he might have known that hands-on work with animals would sustain his motivation to finish.

Gina didn't have a lot of confidence in herself after her attempt at nursing education, but the questionnaire revealed personal qualities of caring/empathy, hard worker, problem solving, sense of humor, and extraversion. The results confirmed that she was good with children, and her mother, who had always been supportive, agreed wholeheartedly. Together they started talking about possible helping-profession jobs. Gina realized that she could continue to work with children and see an immediate payoff in going to school part-time in an early childhood education major that she knew she had an aptitude for and satisfied her desire to help others. Her employer's financial support only added to her desire to pursue this career.

Jayden realized he loved writing that challenged his analytic skills and that had been the appeal in his major. English lit had been a vehicle for his skill set, but he couldn't see a real-world financially viable job that would value these skills. His initial motivation for taking the technical writing job was as a means to a financial end. But he quickly realized that although the content was very different, his ability to analyze and explain complex material played to his interests and skills and presented him with a new world of information to understand and translate.

Jonas

Given a slight nudge from his mother, Jonas completed the GTKMQ, with a tentative goal of a career in cybersecurity. Let's review his answers to some key questions with his tentative goal as a context. In his spare time, along with spending time with friends, he enjoys playing video games and using the computer. He sees himself as honest and hard working with good coping and problem-solving skills. Jonas tried and liked skydiving, so this suggests that he

has a sense of adventure and enjoys a challenge. He wants to develop an expertise in computer security, and his best subject in school was science.

Ultimately Jonas sees himself in a technical job that involves problem solving, using community college as a first step to continuing his college education.
So far, nothing in his responses suggests that cybersecurity is a bad fit. But he
still has doubts about moving ahead.

"So whaddaya think? About the questionnaire thingy?"

*"The questionnaire thingy . . . Oh! Oh yeah, that; yeah, I did them;
you can take a look if you want."*

"And?"

*"Well, you'll see—I mean it's not like I'm running to apply for a
school program or job application because of it. But it did help me shake the
branches and clear out some of the cobwebs and stuff out of that part of my
head. Maybe I was in a rut a bit, I'll admit it."*

"But you think you worked all that stuff out, huh? That's great!"

*"Well, I mean in a way it helped, Mom. But I'm also a little worried.
It's hard not to look at the results and wonder if they're telling me everything
or nothing about what I'm supposed to do. Like the direction that they're
pointing me in, I'm not necessarily sure I have the discipline to commit to it.
I'm not sure that I have the skill sets I need, I guess."*

*"Well, okay, but don't you feel like at least now you're asking these
questions, where you weren't before? I mean I know it might be daunting,
Jonas, but you can pump the brakes a little bit—this is just a starting place,
something to work with and brainstorm on and then move on from there
to figure out how to work on some of these things. I have a few ideas that
might be useful. But I think the goal was to get you to start posing some of
those questions to yourself, at least getting them down on paper and beginning to hash out where the options and pathways are that you're looking for.
Make sense?"*

*"Yeah, Mom, I s'pose you're right, I do feel tentative, but before I was
more just ignoring most of this stuff, so it's good to see it laid out like that."*

Ten days later . . .

*"J, did you grab milk at the store? I sent you a text letting you know
we're out."*

"I did. I meant to. I will now."

"Aha, well okay, as long as it isn't too much trouble. But before you go,

can we talk about the questionnaire? It's been about 2 weeks, and I felt like there was some momentum there, and now I don't know where we stand. Have you thought any more about this stuff?"

Jonas put down his keys and slid onto a stool. "It's only been a little more than a week, Mom. But I mean I have, somewhat. I thought about what we were talking about and the questions. And I have been thinking more seriously about the IT stuff, at least with regard to where I'm at now. Obviously, it would mean going back for some sort of school or training. And obviously I don't have the resources to pay for it. And like with the questionnaire, I think it was encouraging, but I'm still nervous. I'm not an expert with computers, but I think I'm pretty good. And I did check out this cybersecurity thing. It's like 20 credits I'd have to get and—"

"Oh, really? That sounds fantastic. Who offers the courses? I'd love to take—"

"Mom," Jonas tapped his fingers on the counter, "stop, please, just let me finish, okay? This is what I'm talking about. Just, if you want to hear about it, fine, I'll try to fill you in on what I'm thinking. But just don't take it over. Let me just put it out there, and then you can go think about it for a bit and then tell me how you feel."

"Okay, okay. That's fair."

"So it's like a 20-credit program. And I think it works for me, for what I'm like, since I like the computer stuff, it's an exciting and growing area, I can make some money, and I don't have to interact with too many people. Not that I hate people, you know, but just from the questionnaire and remembering working at the department store during high school, helping customers all day, not my favorite thing. But I am worried, beyond just the school stuff, that it's too independent. Like I always worked best when I had a place to go for work and a time when I knew I would be there. Remember when I did legal transcriptions for a bit, online? I fell apart. Everything else on the computer was a distraction, and then I did everything an hour before the deadline. It was a mess. So I'm worried that I could get to that point with this, 'cause they say some of the work is like contracting and freelance almost."

"Yes, that may be true. But Jonas, I think that's putting the horse before the cart a little, don't you? I'm sure you could find jobs that would suit you, and if you're good at it then I can't imagine people having a big problem with you wanting to come into work. Plus, you'll change over time; you'll get better at that stuff if you work at it. I can tell you that I was certainly not the picture of organization and time management when

I was your age. But you work at it and take on more of it over time, and eventually you realize that you're doing a lot more of it without even really thinking about it."

For Jonas and his mother, completing the questionnaire has been a catalyst to engage in a more concrete exploration of the goal of cybersecurity. In that sense, he has progressed from where he was a month or two ago. But Jonas also filled out the Executive Skills Questionnaire in Step 1, and now he and his mother have a better understanding of why he dropped out of college and had a hard time with jobs like the transcription gig that proved to require too much autonomy. Jonas's executive skills weaknesses in task initiation, sustained attention, and time management make it difficult to generate his own deadlines and efficiently produce work.

Jonas may not love his job at the warehouse, but he's found it okay for now and really feels no burning need to move on. Before the GTKMQ, he had little idea what he wants to move on to, and so he's fairly comfortable where he is. Were it not for his mother's impetus, he might remain so indefinitely. When she raises the issue, he doesn't disagree with her assessment or the need to find some direction, but she does have to keep at him.

Completing the questionnaire is a first step but not the be-all and end-all. Jonas is clear that the results of the questionnaire, while informative, have not "sealed the deal." He continues to have some doubts, both about whether the choice is right for him and about his ability to succeed.

Besides serving as a discussion catalyst, the responses yield important information. In Jonas's case, none of his responses suggest that his goal is a "bad fit": he has the relevant interests and basic skills. We also know something about what setting and type of work would not be a future good fit. His experience in customer service confirms that Jonas would prefer interactions with computers to dealing with "people problems."

Another important piece of information involves school. Since cybersecurity school might be necessary, Jonas is clear that it needs to be the quickest, shortest route possible, focusing only on what he is interested in. If your young adult has struggled with school, but needs to return to some type of schooling to meet a goal, this type of information is critical. The school issue for many young adults, as it is for Jonas, relates to the courses required for a degree and the accompanying time commitment. We often see young adults, like Gina, who must take a significant number of required courses in which they have no interest and have no obvious and immediate relation to their goal. They frequently struggle or fail and eventually leave school. Limiting the time commitment (like

Jonas), and taking only courses relevant to quickly reaching the goal, is likely to be more successful.

An associate's degree or certificate programs could be a first step, assuming that the young adult can develop a goal that lends itself to entry-level positions that don't initially require a bachelor's degree. Even if the young adult is not positive this is the right direction, the abbreviated approach offers at least two benefits. It is a way to "try out" an interest area without an expensive and long-term commitment, and it provides a path out of a current job that is a dead end in terms of interest. Taking courses that will maintain the young adult's attention is key. We also know that Jonas needs more external structure to initiate and stay on task (we'll discuss this issue further in Step 4).

In the following section we'll present three more young adults we've met who have been stuck and have now completed the GTKMQ. For each, we'll summarize the key information from the questionnaire rather than reprinting all of their responses. And we'll highlight the factors in their responses and in their discussions with parents that may arise to assist you and your young adult in embarking on this journey.

Cheyenne

Cheyenne, 23, is living at home and working as a bartender. She's earning good money, has a reliable job, and plenty of time to see friends and work out. Other than living at home, Cheyenne is self-supporting. She's not feeling a lot of parental pressure to move out, but it does come up in conversation with her dad from time to time. While comfortable, Cheyenne herself is feeling a bit stuck, especially as she has seen a lot of her friends moving on. She left college midway through her junior year, feeling like she was just drifting through it with no real direction she was committed to. And over time she realized that she had the ability to manage school but couldn't get herself motivated, and her grades steadily dropped off. Cheyenne's executive skills profile indicated weaknesses in planning, goal-directed persistence, and sustained attention.

Cheyenne's dad has the GTKMQ and sees her struggling a bit, but he knows her well enough to think she'll find it insulting if he asks her to fill it out. In a series of casual conversations with his daughter using the questionnaire as a template for himself, he finds Cheyenne able to clarify what she is most interested in, which turns out to be travel and living overseas, for at least a time. She has seen the U.S. State Department in the news, and she thinks working for the State Department would be interesting. But when she looks at their website, she realizes that she needs to finish school, take some courses that don't appeal to her, and, given the competitive nature of the job, would have to do well. In addition, she would need to be knowledgeable about politics and probably learn a language, which seems like pure drudgery to her.

If Cheyenne has an interest in addition to travel overseas, it's in psychology and people. She and her dad discuss different options. Marketing comes up, and she feels that this might be an option. Cheyenne also sees a "Be all you can be" commercial about the Army. This never crossed her or her dad's mind before. But it piques her interest since it could allow her to travel, maybe find an area of interest, and maybe finish school without additional loans. Privately, her dad isn't excited about this, but he doesn't want to discourage her, and it might fit with some of her interests. They agree to begin more specifically mapping out both options.

Like Cheyenne, some young adults won't have an already identified job or career that they are interested in, at least that they are aware of. But the questionnaire yields information about interests as well as skills that can help initiate some brainstorming. Recognizing her interest in travel overseas and her people skills, Cheyenne's initial U.S. State Department idea fits in one sense, but she immediately recognizes the school work required makes it a nonstarter. Marketing could be a fit, but she still seems less than enthusiastic about the prospect of more school.

If your young adult has left college with a less-than-favorable outcome before graduating, the likelihood of success in returning full time depends heavily on (1) school being the only path to a career she is highly motivated to pursue and (2) the young adult having the necessary executive skills, including planning and time management, task initiation, sustained attention, response inhibition, and metacognition. Significant weaknesses in one or more of these sills does not automatically spell failure, but it does necessitate a plan for the accommodations we will discuss in the next chapter.

Regarding her interest in the Army, on the face of it this possible choice satisfies Cheyenne's interests and appears to be a good fit. The Army offers a shortcut to what could be an interesting

> **Ask yourself:**
>
> - *Is the young adult's motivation strong enough to help her complete any necessary education for this career?*
>
> - *Does the young adult have the necessary executive skills to manage the demands of school?*

career choice, the potential for completing school without loans, and perhaps a path to a civilian career. It also potentially addresses her executive skills weaknesses in that the path to the goal is faster than school and action-based, hands-on training decreases sustained attention demands. Her father wisely chooses to help her explore this option, exemplifying keeping an open mind and respecting the direction that the young adult chooses.

Trafina

Trafina, incorporating the advice of her high school commencement speaker, pursued her "passion" in college, majoring in art. After graduating she accepted a position with City Year working on creative projects with disadvantaged teens in a large city. She enjoyed the experience but realized that big city living was not for her. She also needed to find a way to earn a living. Trafina moved back home and applied for the few art teaching jobs that were available but found out that since she wasn't certified as a teacher, she would either have to return to school or look for something else. Money for school was an issue, but she also wasn't sure she wanted to be teaching six art classes per day for students ranging in age from 6 to 14. She had done substitute teaching on and off for a year and had some less-than-pleasant experiences. And, given the few teaching jobs available in art, even if she could get past the school and kid issues, a job in the field seemed like a long shot. She was willing to consider other options but had no clue about what she might do. She hadn't given it much thought in college, where her focus was on the college experience and doing what she liked.

Trafina talked to her mom and dad about it, and collectively they thought the GTKMQ would at least be a starting place. When Trafina finished, it concretely confirmed what she felt was an accurate self-portrait— she was an optimistic and dependable person with an imaginative, creative bent who liked problem solving, as least as it applied to the arts. Visual arts were naturally a strength, but she hadn't thought about her tech skills in this area, which she had honed in her college program. She liked working with others and, given her druthers, would work for a small company doing creative things.

For Trafina this was an interesting exercise, but she still couldn't see a direction. Her mom knew that Trafina was the type of person who could readily focus on a path she had chosen but that seeing other options or changing direction was not her strong suit. The Executive Skills Questionnaire in fact confirmed that Trafina was strong in sustained attention and goal-directed persistence, but weak in flexibility, metacognition, and planning. She and Trafina had a good relationship, and she had in the past helped Trafina through transitions and new directions. Her mom saw some possibilities in Trafina's responses to the questionnaire, but she didn't want to drive the process. Instead, she suggested to Trafina that they Google "careers for art majors." This yielded a variety of options that Trafina had never considered. While she still didn't have a direction, she did have possible choices to explore with her parents.

Trafina's situation presents a different set of issues. She has good focus when she is interested in something, in this case art, but she didn't think about what might come next. She is certainly not the only young adult who is in this position. We would not suggest that young adults abandon their "passion," but if young adults graduate from college with a degree that does not have a clear career path or if the career path they envision has very limited possibilities, they may get stuck, a condition that can be aggravated by the extent of their accumulated college debt, and lead to a longer period of living at home than either the young adult or his or her parents envisioned.

For the young adult and the parents, the steps of completing the Executive Skills Questionnaire and GTKMQ are essential. Young adults who are weak in planning, particularly longer-term planning, and flexibility are much more susceptible to becoming and remaining stuck in this type of scenario. Fortunately, if parents and the young adult have established a collaborative relationship, parents can play a key role in helping to develop and support improvements in these executive skills by engaging with the young adult in the planning process. We will offer more on this issue in Step 4.

> *Weaknesses in long-term planning and flexibility often get young adults stuck in a specialized interest without thinking about what comes next.*

The GTKMQ can help kids like Trafina identify other possible areas of interest, preferably related to their college major and passion. However, if nothing obvious emerges from responses related to their degree, the next step is to identify other interests that could lead to a potential career. This might be in an area of talent, as in the case of Trafina with technology. But it is also useful to look more broadly at responses in the areas of spare-time pursuits, preferred working conditions, and previous preferred jobs. This information can serve as a catalyst for discussion and brainstorming. The parent's role in this situation is to point to resources that the young adult can explore, as Trafina's mother did with the Internet, rather than to be the driver or director of the process.

Casey

Casey, age 25, is living at home and has been working as a teaching assistant (TA) in a public middle school for almost 3 years. He went to college for nearly four semesters, starting his college experience with a vague idea about being a physician's assistant. For the time he was there, college wasn't a disaster, but he partied, didn't like taking gen ed courses, and never quite settled on a major since the prerequisites for a physician's assistant looked pretty daunting. On a downward slope, he failed a course and left with barely a 1.9 GPA. He moved back home and bounced around in miscellaneous part- and full-time jobs for a couple of years and then found the TA job. The job doesn't pay great, but he's not paying rent, only occasionally has to contribute for food, and has a beat-up but drivable car. A lot of his high school friends are around, so although Casey doesn't plan on this being his career, he likes the job and life isn't bad. His parents are getting impatient, but Casey isn't sure where to start on a plan. To get the process moving, they all agree that the first step will be the GTKMQ.

Although Casey hasn't given it much thought since college, he realizes in his responses that he still has an interest in health care. Helping people appeals to him, which explains the "fit" with his present job. At the same time, the thought of extended schooling does not appeal to him. He also would like to be working toward something more substantial, but he doesn't see himself as a teacher. He puts the health care idea out to his parents and, to his chagrin, they immediately seize on it. They think his original idea of physician's assistant or nurse is great since it's a growth profession, the pay is very good, and it offers long-term security. To try to dial this back, Casey presents some reality checks—getting into school given his past performance, time needed to complete school, cost and who pays, and his "hands-on" learning style. They acknowledge that these are significant issues and actually are impressed with his realistic analysis of himself and his situation. They agree to help him explore options that start with where he is now and some next small steps he could take to flesh out this goal.

Casey, like a lot of young adults, went into college with the academic ability to succeed and at least a vague idea about a career that matched his interests. And, like a lot of young adults who eventually get stuck, he didn't have the "self-discipline" (read *executive skills*) and fell prey to the distractions and temptations of the more immediate college environment. If Casey had entered college with a strong interest in becoming a physician's assistant, this could have helped.

Since the goal was fairly far off into the future, Casey also would have needed to see that the small steps of daily college life—performance on tests, completion of papers—had a direct relationship to reaching his goal. When the time horizon for an event extends well into the future, in this case years, for Casey to see what he did in the next 6 hours as important to that event would require strong goal-directed persistence, an apparent weakness for him at the time.

This raises a number of considerations for parents (see the box below).

CAVEATS FOR PARENTS

1. *The young adult's interest in and selection of the goal is key.* Unless you and the young adult are in total agreement on the goal, the likelihood of failure is in direct proportion to your insistence on choosing your son or daughter's direction.

2. *Don't look too far ahead.* Especially when the young adult hasn't had much success with previous goals, very distant ones will feel daunting. After filling out the Executive Skills Questionnaire and the GTKMQ, Jonas is thinking certificate program, but his mother is still pushing associate's degree. For Casey, a small step could be certified nursing assistant or LPN, where his parents are initially thinking RN or physician's assistant.

Small, incremental goals limit the length of the time horizon, the amount of time it will take to reach the goal, and satisfy the young adult's need/desire to experience quick progress. For young adults who are stuck and have failed at a goal in the past, short time horizons make good sense. When the path to the goal is short and the actions needed to reach the goal seem more directly related to that goal, persistence is easier. This also allows the young adult to test out an interest without making a long-term commitment.

> *Start thinking in terms of short time horizons to increase the possibility of success.*

What about You?

What have you learned from the GTKMQ? How has it enhanced your understanding of how your child has gotten stalled, on top of what the Executive Skills Questionnaire has revealed? In many cases the results of the two questionnaires dovetail: The young man who decides to be an accountant because he can make money at it but doesn't have the patience to get a business degree and has only been picturing what he'd do with his income while forgetting to picture whether he could endure spending the entire workweek crunching numbers. The young woman who wanted to live on a farm because it sounded so idyllic . . . until she realized she had no idea if she had the skill set for farming or what it was like to tolerate living 150 miles from the nearest city. The young adult whose singing videos on YouTube have gotten thousands of hits but didn't feel like taking voice lessons or studying other aspects of music—and now has no idea what avenues could channel that musical talent outside of a career as a performer.

Have you been able to get a conversation started on where goodness of fit between your young adult and a goal might lie?

Colin

The following is a "real-time" example of the way that this process can play out. In 2015 I asked Colin to imagine how he might have responded to the questionnaire, had we had it, when he left Nantucket in 2011, which was a pivotal event for him.

> In April 2011, toward the end of 2 years on Nantucket, burnout was creeping in, the solace in the work and isolation dissipated. I had told myself for a long time that my choices were of my own volition, but at the end I had failed; I hadn't graduated, and fled from the shambles of an academic career to hide. The following spring, I wasn't sure what I wanted to do, but I left. I had no eureka moment. I still don't know for sure if I made the right choice.
>
> But whether I made the "right" decision is only relevant to how thinking about the process can help me now. I'm 28, not married, no kids, still turn in late homework assignments, still borrow money from my parents. If I had stayed on the island this entire time working, I'd have $100,000 by now (I know some who did). But I'd still be wondering if I did it because I had to, not because I wanted to.
>
> My dad asked me how I would have filled out the questionnaire at that age, and I imagined it again and again in a more casual, daydreaming way, with daydreaming results. But I think the questionnaire would have pointed me away from continuing what I was doing. And I

think that reflects how I felt at the time: my peers had escaped to the island; I was still escaping from the outside. By comparison, I think I found some R&R from my own self-destruction, had a chance to work, have fun, pay bills, go grocery shopping, and plan a vacation. It helped me reattach to habits I lost track of or never had to begin with. But I wanted to go back and do it again, differently, even if I didn't quite know what 'it' is. So in going "off-island" permanently, I wasn't setting a course for a specific goal, but removing one that wasn't what I wanted. It wasn't only leaving an environment, but also leaving behind ideas about work and a lifestyle that always felt like a shirt that looks great but never fits right. Nantucket was my lab, and I'd gotten some promising results, but I knew that without a field test the results would always feel hypothetical.

Back at home from Nantucket, Colin moved from job to job, but in the process he did narrow his track and move closer to work and interests that require more mental than physical exercise. He does occasionally borrow money, but in terms of both finances and life skills, he manages his own life. I've learned to accept that it is not a quick process and that time is not the most critical measure. Rather, it is self-sufficiency and movement forward on a gradually more defined path and a narrowed range of goals and outcomes.

> *Trial and error are an important part of the process of achieving independence, so parental patience is paramount.*

In this experience, we learned that for parents there are a couple of key points as they go through this process with their young adults. In the path toward independence for many young adults, trial and error are an important part of the process, especially when they have executive skills problems or they've lost confidence due to a lot of false starts toward self-sufficiency. Through a process of elimination, the dead ends are cleared out. And that means that patience, in spite of the anxiety and frustration we can feel, is essential. The take-home message in this step is to follow your young adult on her journey, help her get up and dust herself off when she asks, and encourage her on her way. In the young adults and parents we've worked with, this method has paid off time and again. You'll see but a small example of this in Colin's epilogue. The other lessons we've learned personally and that Peg and I have learned professionally are the subject of Step 4.

STEP 4

....

Plan How to Help—and Where Not To
Parents' Executive Skills
and Respect for Boundaries

"Ceci, you've got to do something about your room—there's stuff everywhere! I don't know how you can find anything!"

"Mom, step back, take a breath. Keeping track of my things isn't an issue for me."

"Well, maybe, but it's an issue for our—"

"Hang on, when my company relocated overseas, you and Dad suggested I move back till I found a job so I could save some money. Made sense to me, we talked about privacy, and you said you understood, right?"

"But—"

"And I'm working, saving money, covering my expenses, and managing my own stuff around the house. Add to that cooking a couple of times a week for us, yes?"

"Well, yes."

"Right now, room cleaning is not the priority; working and getting my financial planning certification is."

"Then just let me help! I can't stand seeing it the way it is!"

"Well, there's your solution."

"I don't get it, so you want my—never mind, just got it."

"Any mail for me?"

"Yeah, Desh, wanna guess what?"

"Tax returns!!"

"It's August. Try a student loan notice and what looks like a credit card statement. Which, by the way, we're getting daily calls from your credit card company about late payments. You've got to take care of this stuff, Desh. Your credit rating must be in the tank!"

"So what? It's not like I'm going to buy a house anytime soon."

"It could affect whether you get a job."

"I'll cross that bridge when it comes. You're being vicarious-miser Mom again."

"Dad! Guess what!?"

"Lemme guess, Shan. Ah . . . okay, I give up. What?"

"I found a car . . . one that I can afford!"

"Hmmm, what is it?"

"A Hyundai, 2008."

"How many miles?"

"Hundred twenty-five thousand, and it's in great shape, and bes—"

"Price?"

"$4,795!"

"I don't think it's a good idea, Shan."

"God, I knew it! When's the last time I had a good idea as far as you're concerned!? I got the Carfax, stayed in the price range you suggested, but that's not good enough!"

"Now hang on. Those aren't the only things I suggested. The mileage . . ."

"It's gotta be your way, doesn't it, Dad?"

"Well, at least we need to talk about it."

"No, not this time. You know what? My money, my decision. I like it and I'm getting it."

"Well, good luck then, Shan, but if that's the way it's going to be, when it breaks down, don't come crying to me for help!"

"Trust me, hell will freeze over first!"

Some of the scenarios above may sound familiar. Friction is a fact of life for circumstances involving parents and grown children sharing a living space, often exacerbated not only by general frustration and impatience but also by clashes over styles of executive functioning. Step 4 is intended to give you and your young adult a window into these differing expectations and some strategies to address them.

In Step 2 you saw how divergent notions about the meaning and signs of independence can halt a young adult's progress, sometimes without young adults and parents knowing they're operating from different assumptions. We discussed assumptions about motivation and readiness for change too—how parents can believe "Of course you want to move out and start your own life!" where their son or daughter may not even know how to take the first step, how parents can give mixed messages about what they want the young adult to do, and how young adults can end up too comfortable or too nervous to leave their current living situation behind.

Step 3 may have uncovered the flaws in other assumptions you and your young adult hold. The results of the GTKMQ often reveal that parents' ideas about what their children can do with their lives, want to do, and are equipped to do are more fantasy than reality. The questionnaire can also force young adults to see that some goals are actually pipe dreams because too many limitations stand in the way of reaching them. Fortunately, at the same time, the questionnaire reveals what *is* possible and can get both young adults and parents started on fruitful conversations about a new goal that is exciting precisely because it is achievable and reflects what the young adult truly wants.

In our coaching work with young adults and parents, we've found that unexamined assumptions are often at the center of false starts and demoralizing detours. Articulating unspoken assumptions and letting them go when they're not serving the goal of gradual independence can be tough for both parents and their grown children. In our experience the key to wiping away unconstructive notions and getting on the same track is communication. That's the core of this chapter.

You want to help your child launch. But do you know where you can be of the most help? That may depend in part on how your own executive skills compare to the young adult's. To give an oversimplified example, if arguments erupt because your son keeps getting sucked into social media instead of searching for jobs online, but you have to push aside a tower of unopened mail teetering on your coffee table to see the TV, you may not be the best person to help him resist distractions. Take the Relationships-Based Executive Skills Questionnaire in this chapter to get an idea of where you can offer the best guidance and support and where you might want to stay out of the picture. In Step 9 we'll steer you to other sources of help if there's no goodness of fit between your executive skills and those of your son or daughter, but most parents we've known find

> *Unexamined assumptions often halt progress toward independence or send young adults and parents on discouraging detours.*

ways to capitalize on their strengths to bolster their children's weaknesses in a productive way. This step shows you how to communicate about that so you can come up with a plan to help. It also shows you how to have constructive conversations about expectations and assumptions and about the boundaries that parents must respect as an essential part of the journey toward independence.

Similarities and Differences That Make a Difference

The Relationships-Based Executive Skills Questionnaire on pages 93–96 allows each of you to directly compare your executive skills with your opinion of the other person's executive skills. That means that if you are the parent, you'll rate your young adult's executive skills, and if you are the young adult, you'll be rating your parent's executive skills. We've found that parents and young adults largely agree on where each other's strengths and weaknesses lie, but bringing this intuitive knowledge of each other to the surface can get you talking openly about the best ways to collaborate.

Before you use the questionnaire, keep in mind that this has nothing to do with comparing overall scores. What you want to look for are areas of difference and similarity in skills; these represent either sticking points or mutual strengths. A big difference is a clue that you and the other person might not see eye to eye on that skill and is a potential point of friction—but it can also be turned into a positive opportunity. Likewise, close similarities are areas of agreement that can be used to establish common ground and shared perspectives, regardless of whether what's shared is a strength or a weakness. If you and your young adult share executive skills strengths, you likely see eye to eye on problems that require these skills. If you share weaknesses, you might have empathy for your shared struggles.

Relationships-Based Executive Skills Questionnaire

Directions: Read each sentence pair and decide which of the two options best describes you. Then decide *how often* the statement is true for you (sometimes, often, most of the time). When you have completed all the items for yourself, go back and follow the same process for the person you're working on the form with—the young adult if the parent is completing this questionnaire and the parent if the young adult is completing it. Decide which of the two statements best describes him or her and then choose how often the description applies. Then look for patterns of similarities and differences between self and other. You'll need two copies of the questionnaire so each of you can complete it; see the end of the Contents for information on accessing the form online.

RESPONSE INHIBITION

	Sometimes	Often	Most of the time	Statement A		Statement B		Sometimes	Often	Most of the time
Self	☐	☐	☐	Carefully deliberates before making a decision	OR	Jumps to conclusions	Self	☐	☐	☐
Other	☐	☐	☐				Other	☐	☐	☐
Self	☐	☐	☐	Thinks before responding; doesn't interrupt	OR	Blurts out without thinking; may interrupt	Self	☐	☐	☐
Other	☐	☐	☐				Other	☐	☐	☐
Self	☐	☐	☐	Gathers all the facts before acting	OR	Acts before getting all the facts ("gut instinct")	Self	☐	☐	☐
Other	☐	☐	☐				Other	☐	☐	☐

WORKING MEMORY

	Sometimes	Often	Most of the time	Statement A		Statement B		Sometimes	Often	Most of the time
Self	☐	☐	☐	Has a head for details (memory like an elephant)	OR	Has difficulty remembering details	Self	☐	☐	☐
Other	☐	☐	☐				Other	☐	☐	☐
Self	☐	☐	☐	Remembers what has to be done	OR	Forgets what he or she has promised to do	Self	☐	☐	☐
Other	☐	☐	☐				Other	☐	☐	☐
Self	☐	☐	☐	Follows through on obligations without reminders	OR	Needs reminders to get things done	Self	☐	☐	☐
Other	☐	☐	☐				Other	☐	☐	☐

EMOTIONAL CONTROL

	Sometimes	Often	Most of the time	Statement A		Statement B		Sometimes	Often	Most of the time
Self	☐	☐	☐	Handles negative feedback easily	OR	Reacts strongly to criticism	Self	☐	☐	☐
Other	☐	☐	☐				Other	☐	☐	☐

(continued)

EMOTIONAL CONTROL
(continued)

	Some-times	Often	Most of the time					Some-times	Often	Most of the time
Self	☐	☐	☐	Is cool as a cucumber	OR	Becomes upset by "little things"	Self	☐	☐	☐
Other	☐	☐	☐				Other	☐	☐	☐
Self	☐	☐	☐	Keeps emotions in check	OR	Gets sidetracked by strong emotions	Self	☐	☐	☐
Other	☐	☐	☐				Other	☐	☐	☐

TASK INITIATION

	Some-times	Often	Most of the time					Some-times	Often	Most of the time
Self	☐	☐	☐	Follows through on obligations without reminders	OR	Needs reminders to get things done	Self	☐	☐	☐
Other	☐	☐	☐				Other	☐	☐	☐
Self	☐	☐	☐	Gets started right away on chores or other tasks	OR	Puts off starting things	Self	☐	☐	☐
Other	☐	☐	☐				Other	☐	☐	☐
Self	☐	☐	☐	Completes tasks well before deadlines	OR	Leaves things until the last minute	Self	☐	☐	☐
Other	☐	☐	☐				Other	☐	☐	☐

SUSTAINED ATTENTION

	Some-times	Often	Most of the time					Some-times	Often	Most of the time
Self	☐	☐	☐	Stays focused on the task at hand	OR	Jumps from one task to another	Self	☐	☐	☐
Other	☐	☐	☐				Other	☐	☐	☐
Self	☐	☐	☐	Once started, keeps working until the task is done	OR	Is slow to finish tasks (or they don't get done)—runs out of steam	Self	☐	☐	☐
Other	☐	☐	☐				Other	☐	☐	☐
Self	☐	☐	☐	Gets right back to work after an interruption	OR	Gets derailed by interruptions; easily distracted	Self	☐	☐	☐
Other	☐	☐	☐				Other	☐	☐	☐

PLANNING/PRIORITIZING

	Some-times	Often	Most of the time					Some-times	Often	Most of the time
Self	☐	☐	☐	Starts the day with a plan	OR	Doesn't plan out the day	Self	☐	☐	☐
Other	☐	☐	☐				Other	☐	☐	☐
Self	☐	☐	☐	Can prioritize when there's a lot to do	OR	Has trouble prioritizing when time is limited	Self	☐	☐	☐
Other	☐	☐	☐				Other	☐	☐	☐

(continued)

	Some-times	Often	Most of the time	PLANNING/PRIORITIZING *(continued)*			Some-times	Often	Most of the time
Self	☐	☐	☐	Breaks tasks down into subtasks with timelines	**OR**	Is not good at project planning	Self	☐	☐	☐
Other	☐	☐	☐				Other	☐	☐	☐

	Some-times	Often	Most of the time	ORGANIZATION			Some-times	Often	Most of the time
Self	☐	☐	☐	Puts things away shortly after use	**OR**	Slow to pick up after self	Self	☐	☐	☐
Other	☐	☐	☐				Other	☐	☐	☐
Self	☐	☐	☐	Keeps personal spaces neat	**OR**	Finds it hard to keep personal spaces neat	Self	☐	☐	☐
Other	☐	☐	☐				Other	☐	☐	☐
Self	☐	☐	☐	Easily maintains organizational systems	**OR**	Has difficulty maintaining organizational systems over time	Self	☐	☐	☐
Other	☐	☐	☐				Other	☐	☐	☐

	Some-times	Often	Most of the time	TIME MANAGEMENT			Some-times	Often	Most of the time
Self	☐	☐	☐	Is good at estimating how long it takes to do something	**OR**	Is not good at time estimation	Self	☐	☐	☐
Other	☐	☐	☐				Other	☐	☐	☐
Self	☐	☐	☐	Completes tasks in the time allotted	**OR**	Has difficulty finishing tasks within time constraints	Self	☐	☐	☐
Other	☐	☐	☐				Other	☐	☐	☐
Self	☐	☐	☐	Arrives on time for things (i.e., appointments, family events)	**OR**	Has trouble getting places on time	Self	☐	☐	☐
Other	☐	☐	☐				Other	☐	☐	☐

	Some-times	Often	Most of the time	FLEXIBILITY			Some-times	Often	Most of the time
Self	☐	☐	☐	"Goes with the flow" when the unexpected happens	**OR**	Is thrown for a loop by unexpected events	Self	☐	☐	☐
Other	☐	☐	☐				Other	☐	☐	☐
Self	☐	☐	☐	Adjusts easily to changes in plans	**OR**	Is upset by changes in plans	Self	☐	☐	☐
Other	☐	☐	☐				Other	☐	☐	☐

(continued)

	Some-times	Often	Most of the time	FLEXIBILITY *(continued)*				Some-times	Often	Most of the time
Self	☐	☐	☐	Changes course easily	OR	Resists changing course	Self	☐	☐	☐
Other	☐	☐	☐				Other	☐	☐	☐

	Some-times	Often	Most of the time	METACOGNITION				Some-times	Often	Most of the time
Self	☐	☐	☐	Can evaluate a situation and figure out what to do next	OR	Waits to be told what to do	Self	☐	☐	☐
Other	☐	☐	☐				Other	☐	☐	☐
Self	☐	☐	☐	"Reads" a situation well to understand the dynamics involved	OR	May be unaware of underlying conflicts, issues, and so on	Self	☐	☐	☐
Other	☐	☐	☐				Other	☐	☐	☐
Self	☐	☐	☐	Is a good problem solver	OR	Looks to others to solve problems	Self	☐	☐	☐
Other	☐	☐	☐				Other	☐	☐	☐

	Some-times	Often	Most of the time	GOAL-DIRECTED PERSISTENCE				Some-times	Often	Most of the time
Self	☐	☐	☐	Sets and achieves personal goals	OR	Is not particularly goal driven	Self	☐	☐	☐
Other	☐	☐	☐				Other	☐	☐	☐
Self	☐	☐	☐	Sets aside immediate pleasures for long-term gains	OR	Lives "in the moment"—takes one day at a time	Self	☐	☐	☐
Other	☐	☐	☐				Other	☐	☐	☐
Self	☐	☐	☐	Sets high standards for self	OR	Is not highly motivated to set high standards	Self	☐	☐	☐
Other	☐	☐	☐				Other	☐	☐	☐

	Some-times	Often	Most of the time	STRESS TOLERANCE				Some-times	Often	Most of the time
Self	☐	☐	☐	Enjoys the unexpected/ unpredictable	OR	Prefers routine and knowing what's coming next	Self	☐	☐	☐
Other	☐	☐	☐				Other	☐	☐	☐
Self	☐	☐	☐	Is at his or her best when the pressure is on	OR	Finds pressure anxiety provoking	Self	☐	☐	☐
Other	☐	☐	☐				Other	☐	☐	☐
Self	☐	☐	☐	Prefers action-oriented or exciting leisure activities	OR	Prefers laid-back leisure activities	Self	☐	☐	☐
Other	☐	☐	☐				Other	☐	☐	☐

How to Use This Information

For this questionnaire, we have three objectives:

1. To see whether your opinion of the other person's executive skills matches his or her opinion. A reasonable match makes it more likely that you'll have common ground for deciding whether a particular goal is a good fit. A discrepancy increases the possibility that the young adult will settle on a goal that you don't think she has the skill set to achieve or that you'll recommend a goal that is a bad fit for her. For example, Jonas has weaknesses in time management, task initiation, and sustained attention, and this gives him pause about school since it did not go well once before. He has a plan to manage these issues by focusing on a small number of courses that are directly relevant to his goal. His mother, however, rated him as stronger in sustained attention than Jonas did. As a result, she suggests an associate's degree because she underestimates his potential executive skills impediments toward that goal.

2. To see where you two have discrepancies in skills. When a parent has a strength in a skill that is a weakness for the young adult, two problems can arise:

- You, the parent, may see the young adult's weakness as an easy fix. You might find phrases like "Let me tell you what I do" or "Just do this!" rolling easily off your tongue. The problem is, easy fixes do not work for weak executive skills.
- When you recommend what seems like a perfectly reasonable and effective solution and it doesn't resolve the problem, you might feel the young adult simply isn't *trying* hard enough:: "If you really wanted to change, you'd put more effort into this!"

Task initiation and time management, in the sense of respect for deadlines set by others, are strengths for me and weaknesses for Colin. From time to time, regardless of the fact that I know, or should know, better, I have heard myself saying some form of "Just do/try this" and wondered if Colin was *really* trying. Fortunately, I've learned, or at least am learning, that these thoughts are unproductive and in fact are an impediment rather than an aid to problem solving. There's also a flip side for Colin and me. When I hear something I don't want to, my reaction can be impulsive and emotional, and I pop off. Colin has a more measured and reflective style and can help me step back and see the situation in a calmer, more rational light.

3. To identify areas where you can offer support to the young adult and where you can't. Assuming you two agree on the young adult's pattern of executive skills, your strength may be a place where you can provide support for the young adult's weakness. From time to time, when Colin has needed assistance with task initiation, he and I have worked out ways that he thought I could help. On the other hand, organization is a significant weakness for me, so he doesn't look to me for help in that area.

How to Talk about the Results

Before you start talking about the results you got from the questionnaire, keep in mind that your opinion of the other person's skills is just that, an *opinion*. So, for example, if you're the parent, show your young adult your Relationships-Based Questionnaire and ask if the young adult agrees with how you see yourself and how you see him. If not, how does the young adult see himself and how does he see you? This opens the door for the young adult to share his questionnaire with you. If you have differences of opinion, the critical point here, especially for parents, is not to try to convince your young adult that *you're* right in your opinion about *his* skills. To do so attempts to put you back in the driver's seat regarding what you think your young adult's problems are and what he should do about them. Such an approach undermines his autonomy and your collaboration. We'll have more to say about the boundaries you need to erect and respect regarding your young adult's growing autonomy later in the chapter.

On the other hand, a difference of opinion does open an opportunity to talk about specific behaviors associated with executive skills. We suggest you start this discussion by asking what behaviors of yours the young adult sees as indicative of weaknesses. For example, Colin could readily point to my study or the fact that I misplace belongings as suggestive of organization issues. Putting yourself first often opens the young adult to thinking about your questions regarding a weakness. For example, I've been able to say to Colin, "It seems like deadlines can be an issue for you. What do you think that's about, or what gets in the way?"

> Try asking the young adult where your weaknesses lie before talking about his weaknesses.

There may be times, even with your efforts to initiate a noncritical conversation about differences of opinion, when you remain convinced that your opinion is correct no matter what your young adult says. If you find this occurring, take a look at how you rate in the executive skill of flexibility.

Not so good? If you can keep this in mind, you might be able to bite your tongue and accept your young adult's perspective on her skills. If her skills later turn out to be a significant mismatch with her goals, you'll both see evidence of this in sufficient time to help with either corrective actions or adjustment of goals. Patience is often essential.

Identifying Similarities and Differences

Now that you've each completed the questionnaire, go back and look at where your patterns align and diverge. A rule of thumb for doing this: *Similarities would be where your young adult's ratings are on the same side of the questionnaire for at least two of the three questions for each skill. Differences would be where your ratings differ on at least two questions.* For example, if under stress tolerance, you selected the *first* sentence for each sentence pair for yourself for all three items and for the other person you selected the *second* sentence for at least two items, then you would conclude that you differ from each other on the executive skill of stress tolerance, with it being a strength for you and a weakness for the other person. And if for any given skill a majority of the sentences you selected for both of you are the same, then you can conclude that these skills are similar in the two of you.

In the spaces below, write down your executive skills similarities and differences. For the similarities column, you may want to note whether the skill is a strength for both of you (place a plus sign next to those) or a weakness (denoted by a minus sign). (We hope you're both using the questionnaire, because the more you work with these tools together, the stronger the collaboration. But if you're a parent reading this book by yourself, obviously you can ignore the blanks for the young adult's results. If you'd prefer to add your thoughts, make your best and most honest guess.)

Parent's Results

Executive Skills Similarities   Executive Skills Differences

_____   _____

_____   _____

_____   _____

_____   _____

Executive Skills Similarities   Executive Skills Differences

_____   _____

_____   _____

_____   _____

_____   _____

_____   _____

_____   _____

_____   _____

Young Adult's Results

Executive Skills Similarities   Executive Skills Differences

_____   _____

_____   _____

_____   _____

_____   _____

_____   _____

_____   _____

_____   _____

_____   _____

_____   _____

_____   _____

Now that you have the results, the two of you can get an at-a-glance idea of whether you do agree on where you each stand on executive skills. If there are areas where you disagree, try talking about them. Chances are such a conversation will reveal some valuable information and you'll ultimately come to agreement. For example, when Colin first suggested that I tend to overreact at times, I pointed out that I had plenty of examples of carefully reflecting on issues before I reacted or gave an opinion. He acknowledged this but reminded me that when I had a strong personal investment in an issue, an impatient overreaction was often the outcome, and he gave me a number of examples. I realized then that he saw the flash point for my emotional reaction and I was able to see my executive skills weakness. On the other hand, if either of you doesn't see the other person's, let those disagreements go. (You can always fill out this questionnaire again after working your way through all the steps, or at some point in the young adult's increasingly independent life, and chances are you'll find that taking this journey together has brought you into agreement on your respective strengths and weaknesses.)

Let's look at what these patterns mean.

Similarities

You and Your Young Adult Share Executive Skills Strengths

Let's start with the good news. When you and your young adult share executive skills strengths, these areas likely are the glue that help you get along with each other. Maybe you both have strengths in metacognition—that means you're both good problem solvers and you both value seeing nuances in ideas, or you appreciate the ability to understand patterns and the deeper meanings of things. Or if you're both high in stress tolerance, you both may be drawn to higher-excitement activities, or you understand why your young adult is. If you look at your shared strengths, you can probably identify how those commonalities make your relationship run smoothly.

How have your shared strengths served you well in the past? It can be instructive to go down the list of your shared strengths and search your memories for examples when these resulted in a good outcome on some goal, individual task, or management of an incident or situation you found yourselves in. Once you've done that, review those examples and see if you can imagine how you could translate that kind of skill application to setting the young adult's goal and/or achieving it.

Jonas and his mother, Marta, share a strength in planning. Once she understood Jonas's reasons for limiting his school expectations, they were able to plan out a course of action together. The plan included selecting courses of interest and a schedule that he could balance with work without being overwhelmed. Together they also worked out the logistics of how Marta could support Jonas's

> The more executive skills strengths you and your young adult share, the more comfortable you probably are with each other, the more interests you have in common, and the more smoothly your collaboration might go.

executive skills weaknesses in a fashion he could tolerate and gave him the best chance of successfully completing the cybersecurity courses.

You and Your Young Adult Share Executive Skills Weaknesses

This is a little trickier. On the one hand, sharing a weakness means you likely understand your young adult's shortcomings, but blind spots can get in the way here. People seem to find another person's shortcomings much more irritating than their own—even when they share the same weaknesses. If you and your young adult are both disorganized, why is it way more annoying when he or she has misplaced something important than when you did?

Colin and I share a weakness in organization of spaces. My study more often than not is a train wreck. And yet, when Colin was living at home, I was routinely frustrated by how *his* room looked, until in frustration he took me into my study and had me survey *my* wreck. After that, my frustration continued from time to time, but I kept my thoughts to myself!

> There is much to be gained—in mutual tolerance and even cooperation at self-improvement—when two adults can acknowledge that they share the same executive skills weaknesses.

One executive skill in particular deserves special mention here. In our experience, parents who are inflexible often don't view themselves that way—but they have no problem seeing their young adult's inflexibility. (See the dialogue that opens this chapter.) For this skill in particular, two people who know each other well may fill out this portion on themselves quite differently from the way they filled it out for the other person. Because one or both of you are inflexible, you could find a discussion about your different perceptions becoming heated. At this point, it might be helpful to walk away from the argument—or crack a joke to relieve the tension. Inflexible people can often see things more clearly after they've had the opportunity to sit with the information for a while.

How Have Your Shared Weaknesses Gotten in Your Way in the Past?

Now try the same exercise with shared weaknesses you listed above. Do a little brainstorming about the instances when a shared weakness created a problem: Do they offer any lessons about what you should watch out for during goal setting and goal achievement? Did your review of shared strengths suggest any ways you could use strong executive skills to avoid these pitfalls?

Colin and I share a weakness in one aspect of time management. While I'm good with deadlines set by others (e.g., the IRS, my doctor and dentist, credit card companies), I struggle with tasks that require self-imposed deadlines such as writing projects and chores. That weakness, for example, led to unrealistic expectations about when we would finish this book and when Colin would complete his undergraduate degree. A shared strength in metacognition has led us both to more carefully project what we can accomplish in a given time. For example, we are jointly working on an interactive coaching platform that Colin will take the lead on over time. Mindful of the work, school, and personal responsibilities he has taken on, we have settled on an 18- to 24-month time frame to accomplish this.

Differences

Your strengths may be your young adult's weaknesses, or your young adult's strengths could be your weaknesses. In either case, the number-one lesson we've learned about this disparity is that if you are naturally *good* at something, it's very hard to understand people who are naturally *bad* at it. If you automatically . . .

- Begin a task as soon as it's assigned
- Arrive on time for any appointment, date, or scheduled event
- Pick up after yourself
- Stop and think before you say or do something
- See a situation in all its layers or from multiple perspectives
- Stick with any task without getting sidetracked before it's done . . .

then there's a good chance you have a hard time understanding why someone would struggle with any of those things. And we may go one step further. While we may be perfectly comfortable saying about ourselves, "You know, that's just something I'm not very good at," when we see a weakness in another person we may attribute it to something that person could control if he or she wanted to. You might find yourself saying, "I'm not good at estimating how long it takes to do something," and then you say to your young adult, "but you're just a slob." Or "I admit I fly off the handle, that's just how I'm 'wired,'" but "your inability to get started or complete tasks—that's pure laziness."

So now that you understand how executive skills can impact relationships, how can you use this knowledge to improve those relationships? Suggestions follow.

Tips for Managing Profile Differences
in Relationships

• **Don't assume that a skill that feels "natural" to you feels that way to your young adult.** If you have an internal clock that runs all the time and calibrates accurately so you're never late and you never try to pack too many tasks into a certain time period, don't assume that your young adult has the same clock. Maybe your clock measures time to the minute and his measures time in 30-minute increments. Or maybe his clock varies, so that 30 minutes feels like 15 minutes one day and 45 minutes the next. Or maybe your young adult has a "close enough" way of viewing time, while you're a minute-by-minute person. Neither one is right or wrong—but they certainly are different!

Through accumulated experience, my wife and I both recognize that "Colin time" is a real phenomenon, and we plan accordingly. (If either of you has been diagnosed with ADHD, you know that your grasp of time is not likely to change, but you may also know that a wealth of tools are available to help. As you'll learn in Step 7, an environmental fix with "real time" measures is a viable option.)

• **Take advantage of your young adult's strengths where you can.** If you have problems with emotional control and it's a strength for your young adult, maybe your young adult should call the credit card company to contest a charge.

My wife and I both recognize and continue to benefit from Colin's advice and management of our disputes with our daughter. He is the "voice of reason" when we can't seem to be rational.

If organization comes naturally to your young adult and it's your weakest executive skill, then maybe your young adult should be the one to maintain the records needed to complete your income taxes every year. This type of reciprocity brings a much more collaborative and "equal" feel to the relationship.

Casey's parents, for example, recognize the strength of his metacognitive skills in his analysis of what is and is not a good career fit for him. Based on this information, they defer to his judgment about the path to a health care career and offer the support Casey judges he'll need.

• **Work on communication skills** (see pages 115–116) so that you can talk with your young adult in a way that shows understanding of your different executive skills profiles. As we've noted, this can work from either side. As I pointed out above, when it comes to father–daughter conflicts, emotional control is not always my strong suit, but Colin's counsel has helped me keep the lid on. Task initiation and time management, on the other hand, are not

Colin's strong suits but, with exception of self-imposed deadlines, they are mine, so for particular tasks like initiation of assignments for courses, he has suggested that I text him at a designated time as a prompt, and this has been effective for him. In both of these cases, our practiced ability to be direct without being critical of one another has made collaboration positive and beneficial to each of us.

Colin's career goal is to become a certified behavior analyst. His weakness in sustained attention, particularly for subjects of less interest, sometimes results in his losing sight of that goal. When that happens, we are able to discuss how a particular course, boredom notwithstanding, directly relates to his more important, long-term goal. The discussion helps him move past what he feels is tedious content.

• **Prepare in advance when an activity involves an executive skills weakness.** If you, the parent, can't—or don't want to—take on the task that uses your executive skills strength and taps into your young adult's weakness, come up with a plan to discuss how he might handle the situation. If he is amenable, work with him on creating a checklist that incorporates a plan and time frame for how tasks that require weak executive skills will be managed. Keep in mind that your young adult does better with small, very specific tasks (wash the surfaces in the kitchen, complete the one-page discussion post) than with larger, more general tasks (clean the house, get a B in the course).

Working toward Identifying a Goal Together: The Relationships-Based Questionnaire in Action

Setting a goal, whether it's to move into a separate residence, start contributing to the parents' home expenses, get a job, or enroll in college or a training course, has to be a collaborative effort between you and your stalled young adult to have the best chance of success. Let's look at how Jonas and others we've introduced started off on the right foot with the Relationships-Based Questionnaire results to inform them.

Jonas

We've suggested so far that Jonas, based on the information he provided about previous problems in college, has difficulties with task initiation, sustained attention, and time management.

The following are summaries of Jonas's and his mother's strengths and weaknesses as identified by them on the Relationships-Based Questionnaire:

Jonas

Strengths	Weaknesses
Flexibility	Task Initiation
Planning	Sustained Attention
Metacognition	Time Management

Marta

Strengths	Weaknesses
Task Initiation	Organization
Planning	Response Inhibition
Time Management	Working Memory

On the Relationships-Based Questionnaire, Jonas's mother identifies his weaknesses as task initiation, time management, and sustained attention but rates his capacity for sustained attention higher than Jonas does, as noted earlier. She agrees that they both have a strength in planning. In discussing her opinion, Jonas explains his sustained attention weakness in the context of his previous college struggles, and she is then able to understand better what got in his way. Jonas identifies task initiation and planning as strengths for his mother and organization and response inhibition as weaknesses. He is able to point out how her quickness to enthusiastically embrace and attempt to extend his school plan to an associate's degree reflects her inhibition issue. He discusses this with her, and they agree that he will sometimes need to damp down her "add-ons" to his plans. We'll see as we proceed through the remaining steps how they use this understanding in goal setting and achievement, but at this point they have a good idea of how to take into account each other's strengths and weaknesses.

Cheyenne: Struggling to Find a Goal

Cheyenne sees her executive skills weaknesses as being in the areas of goal-directed persistence, planning, and sustained attention. She struggles with even identifying a goal, and this likely impacted her college performance since she had no clear idea where she was headed. While this lack of direction in college probably characterizes a number of young adults, many if not most have it sorted out by their junior year when they've selected a major. If not, then they, like Cheyenne, may be headed toward a halt in their development. The following are summaries of Cheyenne's and her father's strengths and weaknesses as identified by them on the Relationships-Based Questionnaire:

Cheyenne

Strengths	*Weaknesses*
Metacognition	Planning
Task Initiation	Sustained Attention
	Flexibility

Dad

Strengths	*Weaknesses*
Planning	Task Initiation
Metacognition	

On the Relationships-Based Questionnaire, Cheyenne's dad sees her weaknesses as planning, sustained attention, and flexibility. He believes that a weakness in flexibility accounts for her difficulty generating a goal, and he rates her goal-directed persistence as higher since he feels that when she has a goal of interest, she pursues it. Cheyenne sees her dad's strengths as planning and metacognition and agrees that they share a strength in the latter.

Fortunately, with her metacognitive skills Cheyenne can identify her interests, and together this gives them sufficient information to brainstorm possible goals. Although her dad has concerns when she identifies the Army as appealing, he understands how this could be a fit for her. With his planning ability, they are able to generate a task list that will give Cheyenne the information to understand the implications of this goal and decide if it still feels like a good fit.

If you and your young adult have a pretty good relationship and you have some information about his interests, *and* if you have some strengths in his areas of weakness, you can brainstorm and plan with him. We'll give some other examples of this below and a more detailed exposition in the next chapter.

Trafina: Roadblocks for Young Adults with a Degree

Trafina has a BA with limited options if she stays strictly within the field of art, and her self-identified weaknesses in flexibility, metacognition, and planning hinder her ability to think outside the box she is in. Her mother, Doris, wisely does not want to drive the process because this puts her squarely back in the parent role and does not help Trafina develop her own executive skills.

On the Relationships-Based Questionnaire, Trafina sees her mom as having the following strengths and weaknesses:

Strengths	*Weaknesses*
Planning	Emotional Control
Flexibility	Stress Tolerance

Doris sees Trafina's pattern of executive skills strengths and weaknesses as Trafina herself does.

Strengths	*Weaknesses*
Goal-Directed Persistence	Flexibility
Sustained Attention	Metacognition
	Planning

Doris discusses with Trafina options such as an Internet search for identifying careers other than teaching for art majors as a first step to broaden her horizon. Her mother recognizes that once Trafina, with her strengths in sustained attention and goal-directed persistence, has a goal that she is interested in she will pursue it with a good deal of motivation.

Four Executive Skills Important to Identifying a Career Path

For young adults who already have a college degree but no clear path to a career, success in finding that path will put a premium on four executive skills in particular. In addition to flexibility, so that they can either try out a different field or find another route besides full-time employment into their chosen field, metacognition, goal-directed persistence, and planning are key. If one or more of these skills are weak, then there may be a need for parents or perhaps a coach to provide support in these areas. Flexibility came into play with Trafina since she had to think about diverse career fields that potentially utilize skills associated with her degree. Metacognition will be called on to help the young adult match her interests with one or more of these diverse career areas. Recognizing her skill in computers helps Trafina think about a possible career in graphic design. Noteworthy here is the fact that Trafina, along with Cheyenne and Casey, relies on the GTKMQ in Step 3 to support metacognition.

Once the young adult has identified a potential career path as a goal, having a concrete plan for how to reach this goal is critical because that plan is used to guide day-to-day behaviors in the service of that goal. Goal-directed persistence, emphasis on *persistence*, is essential since the path to a career may well be longer and less direct than the young

> *For young adults with a degree but no career path, flexibility, metacognition, goal-directed persistence, and planning are key.*

adult would prefer. And, having graduated from college, young adults may have believed that they have overcome the major hurdle to a career, when in fact the real work is just starting. As parents of this generation know, and as young adults are realizing, times have changed and expectations must change also.

Casey: Conditions for Returning to School

In Step 3 we noted that Casey lacked the *self-discipline* to follow through on finishing college en route to his goal of becoming a physician's assistant. Translated by Casey, self-discipline meant he saw his weaknesses in the executive skills of goal-directed persistence, planning, and sustained attention. By comparison, on the Relationships-Based Questionnaire, Casey sees the following patterns for his parents:

Strengths	*Weaknesses*
Planning	Response Inhibition
Goal-Directed Persistence	Stress Tolerance
Organization	

They agree with his opinion of their strengths but admit to confusion about the weaknesses. Casey explains he based his judgment on two actions: their impulsive leap to physician's assistant when he said he was still interested in health care and their impatience and worry about his not moving forward toward independence. While not in complete agreement, they are content to let his explanation ride. From their perspective, Casey shows the following pattern:

Strengths	*Weaknesses*
Metacognition	Planning
Flexibility	Sustained Attention

While Casey was originally interested in health care and becoming a physician's assistant, he didn't map out a detailed plan in terms of the courses and the degree of work required by these courses. So while on the face of it his decision to become a physician's assistant and the start of coursework suggested goal-directed persistence, he could not maintain the significant effort needed to persist or sustain attention in the face of the typical college distractions. We also found out, from his GTKMQ, that he has a more "hands-on" learning style. This executive skills profile suggests that his intended health career path needs to involve a shorter and less-demanding course of study so that the end of coursework and a "real" job are in sight. His parents see Casey's metacognitive strengths in evidence when he explains that health care is an interest that offers good career options, but becoming a physician's assistant is not one of them for him. He needs a more immediate, hands-on option. His parents agree and are able to combine their planning skills with Casey's flexibility to consider the options that will fit with his executive skills and preferences and set a path that will lead to a career in patient health care that offers advancement and good compensation.

In agreeing on a way for Casey to pursue the additional education he needs, while taking into account his executive skills weaknesses, Casey and his parents considered the factors in the box in Step 5 (pages 130–131).

Colin: Translating Goal as Fantasy to Goal as Reality

As we've explained, a young adult's goal will remain an effective motivator only if it's attainable. With the initial selection or establishment of a goal, there is a flush of excitement. As we all do, the young adult sees herself as reaching the goal and thinks how wonderful, how "fantastic" in Colin's words on the next page, it will feel, particularly if it involves significant effort and time. But the motivation provided by the fantasy of the goal is short-lived unless the young adult sees that she is making progress toward that goal, closing the distance. Moving toward and eventually reaching the goal requires goal-directed persistence, which requires that the young adult understand and accept that what she does or doesn't do today can directly impact progress toward the goal. We've also indicated that if the goal is distant, it's critical to establish short-term, interim goals to avoid feeling discouraged by the seeming lack of progress. If, for example, as for Jonas, the goal is to successfully complete five cybersecurity courses, then completing one discussion post by a Sunday night deadline that is worth 5% of the grade for one 8-week course may seem insignificant. The interim goal and the time horizon to reach that goal must then be in sight.

Colin eventually came to the realization that while a goal is important, the goal alone doesn't guarantee success. In a discussion post for a course he was taking, he responded to a quote about "grit," which has been identified as an important characteristic to have if one is to achieve a goal.

> The part that I really connect with in the quote is the idea that it's about doing what you need to do today, before dinner, in the next hour, next 10 minutes. In the past, I subscribed to an educational dream that sounded fantastic as an endpoint, but realized after a long, long time that that dream didn't get me anywhere. I don't really think that much about how it will feel to get my degree anymore; what I think about is what I need to get done for my classes in the next day or two. In this way, I avoid falling into a trap of acting or thinking as if my degree is a foregone conclusion, something that has gotten me into trouble in the past. And I would absolutely credit my repetitive failures with helping me develop a more resilient and measured philosophy.

Colin initially thought the "educational dream" of a degree alone would be enough to sustain his effort. But goal-directed persistence depends on seeing the connection between your actions today and goal attainment. GDP is a weakness for Colin, aggravated by a weakness in sustained attention, meaning if it's not interesting or relevant to him, he struggles to persist. By the time Colin identified a potential career working with children with autism, he recognized a degree was a necessity and saw his weaknesses as an obstacle. Together (we share good metacognitive skills) we recognized this and were able to brainstorm a number of strategies. Adopting the most general major for his BA reduced the number of courses needed and gave him the broadest options for course selection. His executive skills profile favors closed-ended tasks, so we tried to locate courses with objective tests rather than papers whenever possible. And we worked out my use of texts to him to prompt attention, task initiation and completion times, and options for eliminating distractions. We faded these supports over time, and Colin obtained his BA. It is important to note that we both feel that while these strategies were important, the essential key to success was Colin having a goal that he was committed to. But I'm ahead of the story because leaving Nantucket was really the beginning of this outcome.

After he left the island in the spring of 2011, Colin occupied himself with substitute teaching jobs, working with students on the autism spectrum. He had also agreed to work on *Smart but Scattered Teens* and ended up writing all the vignettes. He attempted school online, part-time, with only marginal success, passing one course, failing another. He eventually moved, in early spring 2012, to Boston with a friend and tried to find entry-level jobs, but he was battling a tight job market and no college degree. My wife and I were covering his rent for 3 months. When he couldn't find a job he desired, we gave him an ultimatum to find any job he could in 2 weeks or we would provide no additional help with rent. Almost immediately he found a low-paying but overtime-rich job unloading fishing boats in New Hampshire. Within 2 months, this turned into a deckhand job on a trawler, which is where you met him in the Prologue.

Given what he had done on Nantucket and the fishing job, I was pretty sure he was committed to a career using his hands. We had even talked about his doing union ironwork, since his grandfather and uncle had been lifelong ironworkers and I had done it for a couple of years. Given his agility, confidence working off the ground (he had been a roofer), and practical intelligence, I thought he'd be a natural. But I also saw glimpses of the intellectual need, first in the writing and then in the fishing job, with his interest in the politics of fisheries management.

So from my perspective, while Colin seemed to be drifting from job to job without a direction, he was actually making progress toward independence, particularly as he defined it, and toward what he really wanted to do rather than what he felt he had to do, which was also important to him to figure out. My wife, Megan, and I relied on a few executive skills to keep the process moving. Response inhibition in conjunction with emotional control helped us contain our sense of impatience and time urgency as well as remind ourselves of "Colin time." We also discussed that Colin was working hard to support himself and be independent (3:00 A.M. wake-up time to fish in January, living part-time with his girlfriend, getting us all the fish we could eat!). Goal-directed persistence gave us the willingness to support him when the "one-step back" events occurred (running out of money when they couldn't fish). Our (his and my) metacognitive skills allowed us to realize our shared attraction to problem solving, both intellectual and practical. That's when I had the first glimpse that he wanted something beyond physical labor.

Respecting Boundaries:
If You Want Them to Act Like Adults, Let Them

We obviously were feeling our way along the path toward Colin's self-sufficiency just like any other parents. As I noted, we did try to take into account how we could use our executive skills strengths to support his weaknesses. Most important, we tried to remember at all times (not always successfully!) that it was his life and *his* goal(s) to set. Megan likes the house to be reasonably clean; Colin couldn't care less. After repeated requests with no result, she cleaned his room. He went ballistic about invasion of privacy, and we realized this wasn't a boundary to cross. I worked out a deal to have him give me the trash at the door periodically. My issue came when he went to St. Louis. I pressed him to take any job at all. We had some testy conversations when he refused; he wanted work in education or human services. It took him 6 months, but he found work with kids with severe autism, found a career, and never looked back. It was the reality slap I needed to realize he knew himself and I didn't. As I've said, we had had our own visions for Colin's future as he grew up, and it took time for us, and me in particular, to let them go. And we did so not just because it was a waste of time and energy to chase a fantasy but also because we recognized that *our* vision of a destination for Colin was never going to move him.

If your young adult was honest in the way that she completed the GTKMQ, the information that it revealed may have closed the door on the dream you had for your child's future. How you react to this has significant implications for the support you offer, for the young adult's success, and for the quality of your relationship. Remember Cassie, from Step 2? Cassie's father rejected her goal of moving to a major metropolitan area with a friend whom Dad did not trust. His notion was that moving would be a bad decision for his daughter, and he made it clear that he had no intention of offering her any support. He adopted the "parent" role in his response. In the alternate ending for the conversation, after listening to her explanation and reflecting on his own choices as a young adult, he came around, indicating his *readiness for change.* He adopted a collaborative stance, where, by lending his knowledge and experience, he could help his daughter realize her goal.

Testing Your Readiness for Change

If you say you want your child to become an adult, you have to let her cultivate autonomy. As we discussed in Step 2, many parents profess to wanting their child to "grow up," but then they treat them like kids who need to be protected, they rob them of the decisions that should be theirs, or they give them mixed messages and say "Go out in the world!" while making home so comfy that anyone would be crazy to leave. At this point, are you ready for this change?

☐ Have you been able to greet the revelations from the GTKMQ with acceptance, even enthusiasm, particularly if they don't match how you see your son or daughter's future?

☐ Do you agree with the talents and skills your young adult reported having in the GTKMQ?

☐ Can you keep quiet if the young adult's preferences make you want to suggest something different (living in a suburb vs. a city, getting a job vs. planning a career right now, etc.)?

☐ Have you been able to come to agreement on your respective executive skills strengths and weaknesses after you both completed the Relationships-Based Executive Skills Questionnaire?

☐ Can you accept that you may have weaknesses where you thought they were strengths when your young adult points them out?

☐ Can you resist offering guidance or instruction to "help" with your son or daughter's executive skills weaknesses unless asked?

☐ Have you been able to start talking about possible goal directions using the results of the questionnaires in this step and Step 3?

☐ Have you been able to think about where and how you can offer support based on a realistic perspective on a possible goal direction and your willingness and ability to help in those areas?

Choosing the Right *C*'s: Communication and Collaboration, Not Coercion

In Step 2, we showed a conversation between Chris and his mother in which Chris tells Mom that he has no interest or aptitude for pursuing an MBA degree or career in business. He's interested in computers and social media. His mother not only rejects his choice and attempts to talk him into pursuing an MBA, she also devalues his idea about additional training or a degree even though it is an area where he has both strong interest and skills. And then she makes a subtle but nonetheless coercive attempt to further her objective. Even if her effort was sufficient to push Chris in her direction, he is unlikely to succeed. But if he doesn't follow her wishes and she persists, their relationship will deteriorate and her lack of support for him decreases the likelihood of his success. If Chris completed the GTKMQ and his mother believed what he filled out, she might have understood that she was beating her head against a wall. But Chris and his mother have a lot of executive skills differences, and she has always had a hard time seeing his point of view. Flexibility is not her strong suit, and she's not so great in metacognition either, or she would have learned a bit more from her past mistakes. Fortunately, like most parents, she really does want what's best for her son—what *he* feels is best for him—and so she comes around to his way of thinking and they start afresh on goal-setting discussions. She got a little help from learning better communication skills to avoid coercion (which she was barely aware of using) and lean toward collaboration. See the box below.

PASSING THE BATON
COLLABORATIVE COMMUNICATION TO USE WITH YOUR (YOUNG) ADULT

Effective collaborative communication with your young adult is grounded in the assumption that she has the lead in decision making. The following communication strategies are based on motivational interviewing, an evidence-based approach demonstrating that successful, sustained self-sufficiency is achieved only through self-determination. These are our core *do*s and *don't*s for parents:

Affirm versus Blame

- Do affirm your young adult's abilities and efforts to change: "DJ, you've done a really nice job finding a starting job in construction that matches your interests and skills."
- Don't blame the choice as reflecting a fault: "Once again, you've demonstrated the shortsightedness of your decision making, DJ. Construction is not a real career."

Optimism versus Labeling

- Do show confidence in the young adult's ability to reach his goal: "I think you have the persistence and determination to get that internship, Tevon."

- Don't use a negative connotation to undermine his direction: "Tevon, what makes you think you won't just quit when the going gets tough?"

Reflective Listening versus Expert Opinion

- Do paraphrase or repeat what the young adult has said to convey your understanding: "Siobhan, it sounds like you've worked out a realistic saving plan for your car."
- Don't rely on your advice without acknowledging what the young adult brought to the table: "I think the best approach to getting your car is to get a better-paying job first and then finance it."

Collaboration versus Your Agenda

- Do incorporate the young adult's thinking and offer solution sharing: "So you're thinking you'll take the networking job and start the coursework that will help you move up the ladder. Makes sense to me, Jack. What can I do to help?"
- Listen, Jack, it's a dead-end job without a degree. Take my advice, get a loan for school and get your degree and then job-hunt."

In Step 3, we saw Trafina's mother adroitly avoid making pronouncements about what her GTKMQ results indicated as possible job directions and instead handed over the exploration role to Trafina by suggesting that she search "careers for art majors" online. This put Trafina in charge of what she found out and let her freely respond to what appealed to her and bring up her ideas to her parents, rather than reacting to her mother's proposed routes.

Letting the young adult take the lead is always more empowering than expecting him to react to your ideas.

True readiness for change, as evidenced by communicating in a way that puts the reins in your young adult's hands, is always challenged by this goal-setting process, and the young adult's forward momentum depends on a successful, young-adult-driven resolution. We don't underestimate the struggle this can represent for parents. When Colin decided to quit school and go to Nantucket to landscape, initially my wife and I were both disappointed. Nonetheless, we offered our support, accepted his decision, and decided that whether this was a short- or long-term plan, we would do what we could to help. This move was part of a development process that continues for Colin and us to this day. And it confirmed a point that Colin made for parents earlier: young adults can have short time horizons where ours always tend to be longer.

Shortening the Time Horizon

In one sense, a short time horizon or increment for goals should please parents because it means that the young adult more quickly reaches a new level of independence. So why did Jonas's mother and Casey's parents hope for more in Step 3? Because parents see these goals as indeed just incremental and they would like to see the young adult reach a "better" or more "final" goal. Why? If you're a parent reading this book and your young adult is stuck, you'd probably like to have an end in sight for your parenting role, at least this phase of it. And parents feel less anxious and more like their parenting role is complete when their young adult children are "settled," meaning they've reached certain benchmarks. In the case of school, a degree, particularly one that has a clear career path, is one such benchmark. A follow-on and more important benchmark for parents is stable employment in a job or career field that offers the opportunity for financial independence and advancement. While a more advanced degree might further this end, the key to building independence in young adults is successful, incremental progress in goals they have selected and parental support of these goals.

Your respective executive skills profiles will factor into how you view time horizons. Weaknesses in planning may make it difficult to see far ahead, where weaknesses in response inhibition and goal-directed persistence might make it hard to work gradually and incrementally toward a finish line. Your young adult might be more realistic than you are because when a far-off goal has been set for him (getting a 4-year degree) he's fallen off the rails long before reaching it. If he's had repeated failures to reach long-term goals, can you hold back your far-future dreams for him? If he purports to be aiming for a distant goal, can you think about whether he's just saying that because that's what he has learned you want to hear? How can you work together, using your respective executive skills, to find a good *first* goal and avoid stretching too far? In Step 6 we help you keep time horizons under control by distinguishing between what we call SMART goals (those that can be achieved in a week or two) from what we term milestones (those destinations that can be reached much farther down the road, in 6 months or a year).

> *Remember, where they land is not necessarily where they will stay.*

On the other hand, living at home, maintaining a reasonably comfortable lifestyle, can stretch out a lot farther than you ever had in mind. If your adult child has significant debt (from college loans or other expenses), living at home can be a very viable option, but what initially may be seen by both the young adult and the parents as a temporary safe haven can become an extended and indefinite lifestyle. Since every family situation is different, we're not recommending a specific time frame or deadline by which the young adult moves out. What we are suggesting is that parents and young adults have an open and early discussion about the situation as part of a plan to eventually move forward. This discussion can sometimes be uncomfortable and hence may be avoided by parents and young adults. The result, particularly if parents would like to see some movement and the young adult is not on the same page, can be increasing tension and eventual confrontation, which does not aid the collaboration and planning process. Here are some tips for broaching this touchy subject:

- First and foremost, the discussion doesn't necessarily center on living at home versus not at home. The point is movement forward from where the young adult is starting now. For example, if currently she isn't working, isn't helping around the house, gets up at her leisure, and spends time on social media, moving out is unrealistic. A part-time job or help around the house is the first priority in the discussion. (More on this topic in Step 7.)

- If the young adult has a legitimate reason to be home—low-paying job, high rents, pending job, apartment search, or the like—begin the discussion by acknowledging this as a good current reason and ask the young adult for the next step in the plan or a timeline.

- If parents have legitimate needs—downsizing, location change, new parent relationship, financial burdens—present the need and desired timeline to the young adult and ask for the young adult's timeline or plan to accommodate or collaborate on this.

- If none of these apply, acknowledge lifestyle differences and parent(s)' desire to gradually move on to a new phase in their life.

This presents a number of options for collaboration that will help the young adult gain self-sufficiency, including financial contributions by parents for an apartment, increased contributions by the young adult to home responsibilities, parent assistance with a job or apartment search. Remember that this is a small-steps process toward increased self-sufficiency. Megan and I, for example, gave time-limited financial support for Colin and our daughter, Shannon, and Megan went with Shannon to look for apartments. Remember also that independence involves tasks (apartment expenses, credit, health and car insurance, grocery shopping) that are new experiences for many young adults. Their chances for success are far greater if you're able to work with them on the next steps. At the end of the day, this is a process of support plus limit setting, which reflects what you have practiced throughout your child's development. The key difference now is that you don't have the same control you had when they were younger. What you do control is what *you* do.

The executive skills of task initiation, sustained attention, planning, and time management play a central role in helping to maintain the day-to-day persistence needed to move toward independence from one short-time-horizon goal to the next. These skills are useful when both parent and young adult have them, but if there are gaps, two heads are better than one. The young adult's realization about the importance of short-term behaviors for goal attainment is built on a foundation of emerging metacognition: "If I want to achieve my goal, this is what I need to do today." But simply acknowledging what needs to be done is not, in and of itself, sufficient for the young adult who has experienced failure and is stuck. Good intentions alone will no longer carry the day. For the young adult and the parent in this situation, the next step is the development of a goal that seems attainable and that motivates the young adult, as well as a concrete plan, a road map to the goal. The plan specifies the short-term tasks, timelines for completion of those tasks, and the executive skills supports needed for success. Goal setting and planning are the focus of Steps 5 and 6.

STEP 5

....

Set a Goal

Pull Everything Together and Evaluate Goodness of Fit

Step 5 is the fulcrum for our program to launch young adults and put them on the road to independence. At this point you've gathered all the information you need to set a goal, whether the young adult has something in mind or the future looks like a blank slate. In this chapter, we give you a way to consolidate this information into a summary to evaluate goodness of fit, using one of two forms—one for the young adult who already has a goal or an idea of a goal and one for the young adult who's really stuck, without any idea of a career or other long-term goal, and just needs to set some goal for moving forward toward independence. We'll present plenty of examples from the young adults we've been describing so far.

Evaluating a Proposed Goal for Goodness of Fit

If your young adult, like Jonas, already has a goal in mind, you two can use the form on pages 122–124 (also available online; see the end of the Contents for information) to pull together the information gathered by young adult and parent to examine the goodness of fit between this proposed goal and the young adult's talents, aptitudes, preferences, and executive skills. But first, give a little thought to these questions:

- What do you think right now about goodness of fit between the young adult's personal characteristics and the proposed goal?

- How do you think the goodness of fit between the two of you has served your intention to collaborate with the young adult in his move toward independence?

- Have you learned anything that has started to give you any ideas about a new direction or a new approach in working with and supporting your young adult?

Keep these thoughts in the back of your mind, but fill out the form before discussing the proposed goal.

Okay, this is what we've been working toward, right? Obviously the most important answer in the form on pages 122–124 is whether the goal the young adult has identified or is considering seems to be a good fit for the young adult. If you can say yes, you've got a good start and the answers to the other questions in the summary form become more important.

When the Proposed Goal
Does *Not* Seem Like a Good Fit

If you answered all the questions honestly, and your answer to whether the goal is a good fit was no, you need to go back to the drawing board. What are your options for rectifying a skill or weakness that is the source of the "fit" problem? If there are no options or if the problem involves preference, that points to the need to find a new goal. Here are some possibilities to help you arrive at a decision:

• *Do some parent–adult child brainstorming.* Take another look at the preferences and aptitudes information from the GTKMQ. Do they suggest a direction? (Remember Trafina? She loved art but realized teaching art wasn't going to be for her. The GTKMQ pointed to talent and interest in technology, so she decided to consider graphic design jobs. This capitalized on her art interest and bypassed her aversion to teaching.)

• *Do some research.* The Internet is a vast resource here. Type in virtually any phrase that describes your interests/talents followed by the word "job" or "career" and hundreds of possibilities will pop up. You can start by scanning

Summary Form to Help You Assess Goodness of Fit

GTKMQ

Preferred work situation:

What? _____

With whom? _____

Past work experience:

Like best: _____

Like least: _____

Two talents/skills you have:

1. _____

2. _____

Two best personal qualities:

1. _____

2. _____

Two preferred free-time activities:

1. _____

2. _____

Current educational level: _____

    Major _____

    Interest area _____

What is your goal or what goal(s) are you considering? _____

_____

Does this goal relate to or is it fairly well matched with the preferences and job skills you mentioned above? That is, given what you know about yourself, is it a "good fit" for you?

    ☐ Yes   ☐ No

(continued)

Add any specific thoughts that come to mind: _____

_____

_____

_____

Executive Skills Questionnaire:

What are your two or three strongest executive skills?

1. _____

2. _____

3. _____

What are your two or three weakest skills?

1. _____

2. _____

3. _____

Have your weak skills had a negative impact on your performance in the past?

☐ Yes   ☐ No

If Yes, how? _____

How might they negatively impact your performance on tasks needed to reach your goal? _____

_____

If these weak skills could impact your performance, are you still committed to the goal you have chosen? _____

_____

What are your parent's two or three strongest executive skills?

1. _____

2. _____

3. _____

(continued)

What are her/his two or three weakest skills?

1. _____

2. _____

3. _____

If your weak skills could impact your getting to your goal, could your parent be of any help in supporting these skills?

□ Yes   □ No

If yes, is this acceptable to you?

□ Yes   □ No

Goal: Barriers, Time Frame, Supports Needed

What current barriers do you see that could get in the way of your reaching your goal?

_____

_____

_____

Assuming you will start working on your goal within the next month, approximately how long do you think it will take to reach your goal? _____

_____

_____

_____

What types of supports will you need to reach your goal? (e.g., additional school or training, transportation, living expenses, money for school, tutorial support, executive skills support) _____

_____

_____

_____

_____

_____

them and just jotting down the ones that intrigue you and then narrowing the list to do more detailed research. As in Trafina's case, ideally the possibilities capture some component of your current interests and skills.

It's best for young adults to do this research themselves, but for a young adult who seems to get stuck or discouraged at this stage, parents could take a page from Trafina's mother and just make gentle suggestions of search terms to use. Or do your own research, but be very careful here. You may light on what you think is the perfect career for your son or daughter. But if you present it that way, you've forgotten all the guidelines we've offered for walking the walk of Mom-who-wants-her-son-to-go-out-on-his-own and thus rob him of the self-determination that is a huge part of independence. Read the caveats and *dos* and *don'ts* in this chapter (and review the collaborative communications box in Step 4) to have a constructive conversation on this topic.

• *Plug in a goal tried out before unsuccessfully.* If a goal or direction pursued in the past led nowhere, you might be able to take a fresh look at it in the light of all the summary form information and get some new ideas of directions suggested by the GTKMQ information. Or maybe this earlier goal was just too ambitious but was on the right track. Casey originally saw himself as a physician's assistant, but quickly realized he didn't have the executive skills or desire (at least right now) to complete the required education. But all the data he had collected still pointed to an interest in health care, so he and his parents talked it through and agreed that maybe he should try something less challenging in the field. His parents wisely left it to Casey to research, and he picked licensed practical nurse (LPN) and started looking at how to get the education and licensure.

• *Back off from career and education goals and try using the goodness of fit form for those without a goal* (see pages 122–124). Being immobile for a long time or trying several avenues to independence without success can rob you not only of confidence but also of the mental acuity to come up with a vision of your future self. Start small and build up some modest successes before coming back to this summary form.

When the Proposed Goal Does Seem Like a Good Fit

If the proposed goal seems like a good fit, parents will find some tips in this chapter for starting to think about the details, like the time frame for goal achievement and what supports might be needed (along with ability and willingness to provide them), later in the chapter. The examples in this section may also stimulate ideas of how to start planning, but otherwise you can move on to Step 6 and begin laying out a plan.

Let's take a look at what some of the young adults we've described learned from their summary forms.

• A *good fit takes into account executive skills*. Jonas confirmed that getting certified in cybersecurity is a good goal. His acknowledged difficulties with time management, sustained attention, and task initiation caused him performance problems in college before, so this time around he is limiting the time commitment to academics and selecting only courses in his area of interest, with a clear possibility of achieving a more immediate career payoff.

• A *good fit takes into account current technical skills, knowledge, and personal preferences*. As noted above, if Casey had plugged in physician's assistant as his goal, he would have had to say that it was not a good fit for his current technical skills or his lack of interest in engaging in a long academic pursuit that requires sticking with courses he's not that interested in. But the form did confirm that health care was still an interest, and he could say that going for an LPN license was definitely a promising fit.

Dion's form would have shown that hands-on work with animals was important enough to him to keep him going in a vet tech internship but that even his somewhat strong goal-directed persistence wasn't going to be enough to keep him going through the 7 years of classes becoming a vet would require.

• A *good fit takes into account aptitudes*. Gina thought she wanted to be a nurse because her mother was an RN and she seemed to have a knack for soothing bumps and bruises at her day care job. It turned out that she was a natural at child care, not health care. Taking into account her problems with sustaining attention in courses (like science) that she didn't love made part-time study a perfect way to test the waters and find out whether a degree in early childhood education was truly a good fit for her.

• A *good fit takes into account career preferences*. Good fit, and a feeling of being happily engaged in something you care about, is not all about what you *can* do. What you *want* to do is often just as important. (This is not to say that you have to make a living following your passion or your bliss, because part of adulthood is accepting that bills have to be paid, but what keeps you going— what you're motivated to get up and do on most mornings—is important.) For Trafina, teaching art, on the face of it, would seem to be a good fit with her skills and major. But Trafina is more interested in demonstrating her art than teaching it as a skill to others. Hence, teaching is not a career that she is at all enthused about or motivated by. Her weakness in flexibility inhibits thinking outside the box: she keeps getting stopped by the thought that she has a BA, and shouldn't that be enough to get her on a decent career path? With her mother's assistance, she is able to see other potential careers that appeal to her and capitalize on her art skills. Young adults who are stuck even though they have an undergrad degree face some difficulties that may be unexpected by them and their parents; see the boxes beginning below through page 131.

• *A good fit takes into account the realities of needed support and whether it's available.* Jayden had a problem. He had a liberal arts BA but couldn't see a career path other than teaching, for which he had no interest. Based on his college performance, he knew he had a good work ethic and a talent for writing. To bring in some money, he took a landscaping job while he surfed the Internet to come up with options for a "real job" that fit his skill set. In the interim, his parents agreed to help financially. They paid for his cell phone on the family's plan, for his car insurance, and for unexpected car repair costs, and they put $500 a month into his bank account to keep him afloat, as well as keeping him on their health insurance. When he landed the tech writing job in October, like Jayden, they weren't sure this was going to fit. His success encouraged their continued support for a master's degree in technical writing, and he parlayed this into a high-paying job with a top-notch biotech company in Silicon Valley.

LENDING CLARITY
TO GREAT, BUT FUZZY, EXPECTATIONS: FLEXIBILITY

Unless your young adult's degree is targeted toward a specific career track (such as nursing, accounting, computer science, engineering) where jobs are more plentiful, he may not find a job in a field related directly to his degree (e.g., history, English, psychology, economics, political science). Like Trafina, he may have chosen a major of interest or even passion, but either without a longer-term plan for where this might take him or with expectations of a career in a field where there is, in fact, little demand. This is where flexibility comes into play.

Young adults with no clear career path related to their degree may not be working because they don't want to be in the position of settling for just anything. Or, like some of the young adults we've been describing, they may be employed but recognize that there is no long-term future in their job. What's the solution? Talk it through:

Does the young adult have any background in her purported career preference? Absent a degree that's directly related, has she acquired any experience through an internship, field placement, or previous job experience? This may give her a leg up. In the absence of a degree, Colin's previous experience working with students on the severe end of the autism spectrum was essential in helping him land his first job. The young adult without related education or experience will likely start to realize that she's chasing a long shot if she doesn't become more flexible.

Is her job search effective? We're often struck by the lack of familiarity with effective, focused search strategies exhibited by many young adults. Does the young adult executive skills profile indicate weaknesses in metacognition, flexibility, or planning? If so, the parent may be able to jump-start the process by discussing three or four search resources. If there are specific online links to these, they can be texted or e-mailed to the young adult, but parent help should not go beyond resource suggestions. The young adult makes the choice about whether to use them and which one, if any. If not, there are a variety of resources on the Internet, and college placement services are often made available to graduates of that school.

Is the young adult willing to take an entry-level position in her area of interest, even though the pay is low, or perhaps unpaid, as a volunteer? And if the latter (i.e., unpaid), are you, the parent, able and willing to support your young adult in this process? If you are, we strongly recommend that if the position is unpaid, you offer support for a defined, time-limited period such as 3 months. In addition, you and your young adult should agree that she will continue her active search for a paying job while volunteering.

Can you two agree on a time period for this alternative, after which she has to get a paying job? The GTKMQ may provide clues for areas of interest to explore, but since you, the parents, are footing the bill, this is not the time for her to be choosy or fussy. It's time to go to work because regardless of the job, there will be both tangible and intangible benefits. Finding and keeping a job requires application of executive skills and provides an opportunity for the young adult to demonstrate a good work ethic by being on time, showing initiative by seeking out additional responsibilities, and pursuing whatever learning opportunities the job may offer. Demonstration of these qualities leads to good recommendations for any future job since all employers value these behaviors. The young adult development literature also indicates that one's sense of self-efficacy and self-esteem decline as the period of unemployment lengthens. And there is the more immediate benefit of increased financial independence, which is a benchmark for independent living.

Taking a systematic approach to getting a more preferred job: The young adult needs to . . .

1. Broaden his perspective to look at related fields where his degree skills could be utilized.

2. Eliminate unattractive jobs within those related fields and then look at the jobs, at any level, that are available in those careers that are attractive.

3. Adjust expectations, with a view toward getting a "foot in the door." We know a number of young adults who are certified teachers and have taken jobs as classroom aides or paraprofessionals to build relevant experience and be as close as possible to where teaching jobs might open. As we noted above, in this case it is essential to demonstrate good work-related executive skills that translate into a good ethic. Outside of the teaching area, we also are familiar with a large 24-hour fitness club chain that is routinely trying to hire entry-level overnight desk and cleaning staff. For their management and executive staffs, they recruit primarily from people who have started in these entry-level positions. This practice holds true for many corporations. Thus, for young adults who are sure that they do not want long-term employment in their current job, looking at entry-level jobs in an area of interest may be the best immediate option. However, we also want to emphasize that until they have a firm commitment for a new job, it is essential that they stay in their current job.

DOES COLLEGE HAVE TO BE VOCATIONAL SCHOOL?

We want to be clear here. We are not in any way suggesting that a college degree in an area unrelated to a specific career path is of little or no value. While the economic value of a bachelor's degree may have declined somewhat, it is still clearly the case that over one's lifetime of work, individuals with bachelor's degrees earn substantially more than those without degrees. In addition, there is an undeniable and impenetrable ceiling to employment for those who do not have degrees. Let's take an employment area we are quite familiar with, direct service jobs in education or the human service field (e.g., educational therapist, behavior therapist, case worker). If you're fortunate, the minimum criteria include "bachelor's degree *preferred*," but more often than not they specify "bachelor's degree *required*." And this occurs in spite of the fact that a bachelor's degree may have little or nothing to do with the job in terms of education or experience. Yet the absence of a degree becomes the first exclusionary criterion. Colin's classmates, and Colin himself in his online degree program, cite this barrier to certain jobs, or to advancement within their current job, as a primary reason for pursuing a degree.

In this era of technical and technological jobs, you might be surprised to know that liberal arts degrees are enjoying a new desirability by employers in tech fields. In July 2015 *Forbes* published an article ("That 'Useless' Liberal Arts Degree Has Become Tech's Hottest Ticket") whose points have been echoed in the years since: The noncoders and nonengineers are highly valuable, in marketing, sales, and elsewhere, for their abilities to write clearly, think critically, and figure out what end users of tech products want in their real-world daily lives. As the article put it, "The more that audacious coders dream of changing the world, the more they need to fill their companies with social alchemists who can connect with customers—and make progress seem pleasant."

Could your young adult find a place in this burgeoning new employment environment?

FACTORS KEY TO SUCCESS IN PURSUING EDUCATION OR TRAINING

- That the young adult has freely (without parental coercion) chosen a goal that is a reasonable match with the best information available about his work/academic skills, preferences, and executive skills

- That if there is a degree of mismatch between the goal and the executive skills required, the young adult is willing to work with his parents to determine how the weak skills will be addressed and is willing to accept help from some source (Steps 7 and 8)

- That the parents, to the extent that they are able, will support the young adult in his pursuit of the goal

- That the young adult and parents understand what steps the goal will require and a projected timeline for reaching the goal (discussed in Step 6)

- That a concrete accomplishment of the goal—for example, an entry-level job—be attained in a maximum time frame. What that time frame will be depends on the length of the school program. As we noted in Step 2, in terms of paying for school, it's important for the young adult to have "skin in the game," which means that he contributes to or even covers the cost of school with loans or savings. If parents decide they will finance school, we strongly recommend that this support be continued on a course-by-course performance basis with a performance standard (e.g., grade) established and agreed on in advance. Upon completion of school, since it is career-focused, we think 3 months is a reasonable time frame in which to secure at least an entry-level job.

When You're Not Sure Whether the Proposed Goal Is a Good Fit

What if the tools we've supplied show that the young adult has arrived at a goal that seems to be a good fit but you're still not convinced? Here's where the rubber meets the road and you call on all of your powers of collaborative communication as well as your commitment to supporting independence versus encouraging dependence. There's no doubt that this is tricky ground to tread. As a parent you need to feel comfortable enough with the goal without making your own comfort a condition for the young adult's pursuit of it. If you and your young adult can reach agreement, express it. Before reaching that agreement, resist expressing your disagreement or establishing the idea that your approval is a prerequisite for moving ahead with the goal.

Colin's success at and enthusiasm for the work he was doing in autism confirmed that the area was a good fit. But he knew and I realized from his conversations about the work that for him behavior technician was not a career in itself. In his chosen field, he had creative ideas and legitimate critiques about what he observed, but he lacked status in the accepted hierarchy of the field to have his ideas implemented. That status was granted only to people with advanced degrees and certifications. And for him, that was the rub. Advancement meant a graduate degree, and school has been his Achilles's heel in terms of good fit. He felt like the end result would get him past it, but I felt like his executive skills weaknesses might still be an issue.

When you're not confident that a goal is a good fit for your young adult, discretion is definitely the better part of valor.

Here are some basic guidelines we've found useful for dealing with uncertainty.

Don't Yield to Anxiety

If your young adult is stuck, you likely have witnessed some past failures to attain goals and want to spare him another disappointment by trying to "shore up" the young adult's goal or plan through requests and/or suggestions. You might find yourself tempted to:

- Request chapter and verse on how the young adult plans to reach the goal because you figure if she has thought the goal through, she also has a plan in mind for getting there. Watch out for saying things like this: "So, one more time so I understand, can you give me some details, the specifics, on how all of this is going to work out?" Note the little things in the language you use: This sentence would be bad enough if it had ended with "work," but "work out," while it sounds innocent enough, shifts the focus from the logistics to the outcome and makes the parent's doubt very clear.

- Suggest stretching the goal to a more advanced or ambitious level to make sure it really leads where you want it to go—to a secure and stable future. Here too, it would be very easy to turn enthusiastic support into steering the young adult to your own agenda: "Wow, what a great plan! This could even lead you back to grad school, and then the sky's the limit." This represents stretching the goal, laying the groundwork that grad school is a prerequisite for true success.

- Point out all the obstacles that the young adult may encounter. Don't say "Clearly you've put a lot of thought into this, and that's great because it's going to take a lot more to actually get there, like *a lot* more."

All of these attempts to ease your own anxiety will only put you in the executive, parental role again and thwart the young adult's progress. Hold your tongue.

Accept the Calculated Risk

There's no getting around it: The decisions our kids make and the outcomes of those decisions are not a sure thing. Deciding on whether a goal is *truly* a good fit is a calculated risk for us and our young adults. We can only make our best estimate about goodness of fit and, based on that estimate, whether the outcome—goal attainment—is more likely than not. You can keep the risk relatively low if you consider the potential roadblocks, but at this point that means being aware of them, not sounding the alarm.

Keep It to Yourself

Since our children reached young adulthood, whenever I have been involved in some sort of support role I have struggled to keep my mouth shut and to do less rather than more. As both of our children can attest, whether providing financial, emotional, or executive skills support, I have to be constantly reminded by myself or by them to let them manage the process. As has been the case throughout this process, I've learned that our adult children succeed more often than not. Yes, young adults occasionally stumble and fall. As they would readily acknowledge, ours have. And in every case, bruises notwithstanding, they have recovered, learned from their falls, and moved forward. Most important, having negotiated the challenges, they have learned and incorporated strategies that no amount of "wisdom" from me could have given them. Our role as parents is not to say, "I told you so" or to take over the process. It is to help our adult children, if they ask, to get up, dust themselves off, and start again. It has taken me some time to both realize and learn to live with what I now know is part of the development process. And my professional background did not make this process any less stressful as a parent.

Launching an extensive analysis or evaluation of the young adult's goal can be a real conversation stopper at this early stage. When you're discussing the goal that seems like a good fit, focus strictly on how well your young adult's aptitudes, preferences, and skills match up to her goal. Say "Tell me which of your strengths look like they'll be the biggest help to you in pursuing this goal" instead of pointing to a weakness or gap revealed on the executive skills questionnaire and asking, "How do you expect to be able to get around *this*?"

> Ask young adults who have struggled to find their way and virtually all of them will say they have no regrets because they wouldn't be who they are today without having gone through their own trials and tribulations.

During a conversation with his mother in considering whether cybersecurity is a good fit, Jonas starts talking about his ambitions and how they synchronize with his skill set. "This coursework, it's pretty much right up my alley anyway—a lot of it is stuff I already know, maybe not in the academic way they

> *Going along with a goal or plan while imagining saying "I told you so" when it fails is not support or collaboration.*

want, but I know it." His mom offers a reflective response: "That's great, you already have good experience with the practical side, and figuring out what skills you already have will add to all the knowledge you've already acquired." In this exchange, Mom is essentially paraphrasing what Jonas already said, but also note that she is attempting to drive a little deeper at what she believes *his* core motivation is—turning a beloved hobby into a marketable and enjoyable profession.

Your role is to listen and to make your own preliminary assessment about goodness of fit (and for now, keep your opinions to yourself!) while encouraging your young adult to find his own way. Commit the following *dos* and *don'ts* to memory.

DOS AND DON'TS OF SUCCESSFUL SUPPORT AND COLLABORATION

Even if you're not completely sold on the young adult's choice of goals, keep in mind that our tools are designed to offer assurance that there is in fact goodness of fit—or that it's absent. So your job now is to support and collaborate in the discussion phase and through the planning and goal achievement phases that follow. Here are some tips for staying in this role.

Do

    ✓ Let the young adult know that you are available.

    ✓ Offer advice only when solicited.

    ✓ Ask whether it's okay to offer advice if you feel you really must.

    ✓ Accept that your advice is a take-it-or-leave-it proposition—if the young adult chooses not to take it and you find yourself arguing with him, you've crossed the boundary of his autonomy.

    ✓ Support your young adult's goal if his plan is realistic.

And prepare to do these things once you're in the planning and goal achievement stage starting in Step 6:

✓ Continue to provide support as long as there is evidence that the young adult is making progress on the path that *he* has set to his goal and his accomplishments move him closer to self-sufficiency as defined by measures provided in Step 6.

✓ Provide regular words of encouragement and praise for the effort that your young adult puts in and not solely for the successes she demonstrates.

✓ Start with "What can I do to help?" if your young adult stumbles or falls, beginning the problem-solving process with an outcome that you both agree is fair and moves the process forward.

Don't

✗ Point out why the young adult's goal or plan is flawed and then, with each stumble or misstep, say that this confirms your original opinion.

✗ Insist on your own strategy for reaching the goal.

✗ Deny support in favor of a "tough love" stance, which ostensibly provides independence but is typically designed to force the young adult to fail and return to you for your advice and support.

✗ Make your support contingent on the young adult adopting the goal or plan to reach it that you think is best.

Laying the Foundation for Success: Think Through the Challenges before Planning Begins

Even goals that seem like a good fit for an unlaunched young adult will present some challenges or barriers to success. (If they didn't, the young adult probably wouldn't have gotten stuck to

> Remember, "good fit" does not mean "perfect fit."

begin with.) To get the planning of Step 6 off on the right foot, the two of you need to figure out how likely it is that the obstacle can be overcome. How much time and what resources are available to the young adult? What assistance are you willing and able to provide? Is the goal desirable enough to the young adult to make the costs worth the potential outcome? Being aware of obstacles is an essential first step, to be followed by collaborative problem solving to determine what strategies and supports will be needed to overcome the obstacles and where these supports and strategies will be found.

• *Are the young adult's executive skills aligned with achievement of this goal?* Step 4 gave you the opportunity to talk about executive skills strengths and weaknesses—both the young adult's and the parent's—and undoubtedly stimulated reflection about how any weaknesses factored into failure to meet various goals in the past. But the summary form may nonetheless show that the goal that's a good fit in many ways depends on executive skills in which the young adult isn't strong. In this case, you could discuss three options for pursuing this goal anyway:

1. Allowing the parent to help if the parent is strong in the young adult's weak skills: "Trafina, you said seeing options can be tough for you. Want to take some time tonight to sit down and brainstorm about careers?"

2. Finding ways to modify the task or environment in which the goal will be pursued (usually work or school) to compensate or using some science-backed methods for boosting weak executive skills—these resources are discussed in Step 7: "Hey Casey, you said you'd like to get some health care experience before you start LPN school. If you want, we'll pick up the tab for the 50-hour CNA [certified nursing assistant] course that could give you a leg up."

3. Getting creative and using tools and innovative techniques to address the specific weaknesses that will be a big problem with this goal—these resources are covered in Step 8: "Col, you're better with phone apps than I am. I just got the Windows upgrade and it's got all kinds of time management tools you can access on a phone. I'll spring for the student version if you're interested."

What's important overall here is to find a constructive way to talk about any executive skills challenges that factor into the goal under consideration: "Jonas, you've been up front about the executive skills that got in your way last time in school, and you said that's still in your head. You covered part of this by limiting the time frame to a year and taking only courses that should be interesting and a direct route to your goal. Getting stuff in on time was definitely a thorn in your side before. You said I have pretty good task initiation and time management skills. If it would help and won't annoy you, I can text you to start or finish assignments on due days. And I can show you a couple of the Google tools I use to keep on top of work and you can substitute those over time."

• *Does the young adult have a good grasp of the credentials, costs, and/or time frames that will be required to attain the goal?* The credential and cost issue has become a significant problem for many young adults. Tuitions continue to increase, and with readily available loans, debt has increased. Young adults are susceptible to the seductive marketing pitch of colleges—easily attained degrees and successful careers if you enroll in their curriculum. This can lead the young adult to underestimate the time frames and/or the number of courses required to complete a degree or obtain a certification for some career path (e.g., computers, automotive mechanics, health care, electrical work). We see increasing numbers of young adults emerge from this experience with little to show for it other than significant debt.

One young adult, Cheyenne, correctly identifies the alignment between her interests and a U.S. State Department job. The misfit becomes evident to her when she discovers the number of unappealing courses she needs to take to realize her goal. Marketing has a bit more appeal for her, but college costs remain a significant issue. The Army isn't definite, but it aligns with her interests, diminishes the barriers of coursework and costs, and represents a potential career path.

• *Has the young adult accurately estimated the support or assistance that will be available to fill any shortfalls?* Where will the young adult get any material support (tuition, living expenses, car, etc.) needed? What about academic support if subject-area skills are weak? And executive skills support for weak skills? The young adult needs to investigate all of this in advance of final goal setting, and this most likely involves talking to parents about what resources they are willing and able to contribute. We've seen many young adults enroll in college without ever investigating whether the supports and accommodations they received in high school to compensate for weak executive skills would be available in their new educational institution. We've seen kids snap up a "fantastic" internship that would lead to their ideal job without ever finding out how much it would pay (if anything), how much their living costs would be if they needed to relocate for the internship, or what type of guarantee there was (if any) that a job would be offered to them once the internship was up. We've watched stalled young adults sign rental agreements to share apartments with roommates they've never met—and who ended up bailing and leaving the young adult with the entire rent responsibility. We've seen parents try their best to demonstrate their confidence in a young adult by loaning her money to buy a car she had researched extensively, only to realize they had failed to do their own due diligence regarding maintenance costs for that make of car—which of course necessitated further financial help once the car had been purchased.

Tips for Talking about Challenges

- Ask yourselves: What specific challenge does the young adult and/or parent see?

- Discuss: If there are missing elements (such as a specific skill), what might the young adult need to add or clarify to improve goodness of fit?

- Remember that this is just a preliminary conversation to flesh out the specifics as a first step in deciding whether the goal is realistic.

- Detailed problem solving and solutions are not the goal here.

- The point is to highlight possible barriers to give the young adult and parent time to mull them over without the pressure of coming to immediate decisions and stimulate new ideas about managing the barriers.

- Take care during this discussion to focus on the positives—preliminary problem solving—so that the young adult has no reason to perceive clarifying questions as an attack on or rejection of the goal or an attempt by the parent to take over the process.

- When in doubt, leave it out, as the saying goes. This may seem nitpicky, but if you find yourself about to start objecting to an idea with the word "But," *don't*—and throw the rest of the phrase away.

- Avoid cautionary phrases like "You've put a lot on your plate/This has a lot of moving parts/This is a real mountain to climb." If this is meant as a warning, simply don't say it; it ultimately serves no purpose beyond your publicly hedging your support. If it is meant to congratulate or praise the young adult for taking on such a task and showing initiative, then say that instead: "I'm really proud of you for putting this together." If it is intended to elicit clarifying information about how your child will sort out the details, ask permission beforehand. This sounds silly in the abstract, but it is something we (people in general) do all the time. "Do you mind if I ask you a question?" Then wait for a response; most of the time the answer will be yes, but respecting the answer allows the young adult to retain control of the conversation.

Setting a Goal for Young Adults Who Don't Have One

It's not uncommon today for young adults to remain dependent on parents or other family members for financial support or a place to live for longer than any of them anticipated. Many of these young adults also don't see or are not seeking a pathway to greater self-sufficiency. Each of the young adults we've introduced started in this position. In each case there was some precipitant to movement—a nudge from parents plus the provision of the GTKMQ, an awareness that peers were moving on, the perception of a current job as a "dead end." As we discussed in Step 2, however, powerful forces can leave some young adults unmotivated and unready to move forward, from a reasonably comfortable and familiar lifestyle to the effort required to change. If the pros of remaining dependent still outweigh the cons for your young adult, what do you do? The following examples present some options.

James: A Leap of Faith into a New Job

James is a 24-year-old currently living at home with his parents and younger sister. He completed his BA in English from the state university in 5 years. He has educational loans totaling $17,000. While in college, James's long-term (and very tentative) plan included going to law school. But after graduation, when he considered the additional school time, the expense, and the supply–demand issues for lawyers, James decided it was not for him. He took a customer service job with a car rental company about a year ago. Part of the attraction then was the potential option of a management-training program. But James has found this type of work is not a good fit for him. He struggles attending to the details of work and finds himself easily distracted. Recently he received a written warning for playing fantasy sports during work. He tells his parents that he has decided to quit but he has no idea what he'll do after this. Options?

• James's parents insist that he keep his current job until there is a clear plan to move forward. While there are exceptions (abusive supervisors, dishonest practices, substance use by coworkers), we recommend that the young adult who is working maintain his job until he has a viable next step. At the same time, this option has a limited time span if the job is a bad fit since job performance problems may lead to termination. And in a reasonably decent economy, lower-paying jobs such as this one are readily available. So better to leave than be fired.

• But what moves this forward? His parents, keying in on his early interest, suggest becoming a paralegal. From their perspective, it's a shorter, less-expensive path that still maintains the lawyer option down the line. For James, while the pay might be better, this work is even more detail-oriented than his current job, which could be an issue. In addition to requiring more school, he doesn't see it qualitatively as very different from a current job that has no appeal to him.

• When they all look over his GTKMQ, nothing stands out as a potential "passion." James is reasonably familiar with technology but doesn't see it as a career. He likes to be physically active, works out, plays racquetball, and is in a pick-up basketball league. In his limited job experience, he enjoyed landscaping, but it's seasonal. His parents would like him to settle on a career path, but nothing stands out as a direction. And neither they nor James want a choice just for the sake of a choice that turns out to be a dead end.

• With loans due and his parents still helping with some expenses, James realizes that even though he's not anywhere near settling on a career, he needs a job, preferably one that pays decently. A college friend and fraternity brother he worked summers with started work with a construction company right after graduation. He moved up to a foreman's job, and James contacts him to ask about a job with the company. He friend says they are hiring laborers and the pay is good. Since his friend knows James's work ethic from landscaping, he's happy to vouch for him. The company is always looking for people who are hard-working and reliable.

• The job means moving around, but his friend says they can room together. James, although thinking of the job as a "placeholder" while he decides on a career, finds himself excited about this opportunity. His parents, on the other hand, are not. They wonder about the value and use of his college degree, they don't see construction as a "career," and they are left unsure about his future.

Can this construction job be viewed as a goal with goodness of fit for James? First, note that *James* has chosen the path, and he is excited about the change. In part, his excitement may be based on a "grass is greener" element compared to his present job, but his enthusiasm is nonetheless important. Time will tell, but he did enjoy the hands-on work of landscaping. In addition, on the face of it this type of work is a better fit with his attentional capacity. A second significant element is that in this move James has increased his self-sufficiency by moving away from home and increasing his salary. Admittedly, this type of work is not the traditional path for college graduates. However, employment prospects in the building trades are expected to be excellent in the coming years and college graduates have a leg up for moving into management roles (see the discussion in the box on pages 129–130 about the virtues of liberal arts degrees). So in terms of building autonomy and independence, James's decision meets the essential criteria.

Shayleigh: Becoming an Adult at Home First

Shayleigh, age 25, is living at home with her mother and stepfather. She dropped out of college a few years ago and has had a series of intermittent part- and full-time jobs, none of which have resulted in sustained employment. She currently works 20 hours per week in a clothing store at the mall. The job provides no benefits, but Shay has health insurance under her parents' policy through age 26. Her parents bought her an inexpensive car a few years ago so she could get to work or look for jobs. They pay for her auto insurance and her cell phone as part of the family plan. Shay continues to see a few friends from high school and has an on-again, off-again boyfriend who works for his father's cleaning service when he needs extra help.

Since Shay doesn't have to be at work till 1:00 P.M., she can sleep in most mornings, which suits her since she is not a morning person. She has an active social network on Facebook, which occupies much of her time if she is not hanging out with her boyfriend or friends. The rest of her time is spent watching on-demand shows through her parents' Netflix account. For the most part, Shay takes care of her own personal expenses (clothes, cosmetics), washes her own clothes, and takes care of her room (in a manner of speaking). She does not cook, clean, or shop for the family, nor contribute to household expenses. If asked to help with a task, she usually will agree but as often as not "forgets," so her mother feels like if something needs to get done, it's easier and more reliable to do it herself. Task initiation is not one of Shay's strong suits.

Shayleigh occasionally acknowledges being bored but can usually find ways to entertain herself. In general, she is pretty comfortable with her lifestyle. Shay doesn't see living like this forever, but she figures something will come along that interests her enough to move on. Planning, clearly, is not a priority.

Until now, her parents have more or less just lived with this situation, thinking that at some point Shayleigh will "get it together." And since her husband works a lot of hours, her mother appreciates Shay's company for dinner. But increasingly, Shay's situation is a topic of conversation and sometimes conflict between the parents. In the past her mother has typically

come to Shay's defense, but even she realizes that the situation is not good
for them or probably for Shay. The question is what to do.

• In talking it over with her husband, Shay's mother, although she doesn't relish the possible conflict, suggests that she should probably take the lead in setting some expectations. If her husband starts, Shay is likely to frame it as a "wicked stepfather" issue. But Shay won't question her mother's love, and her mother knows she needs to toughen up with Shay.

Since her work situation is unlikely to change immediately, her mother and stepfather decide that Shay can begin to earn her keep by contributing to family responsibilities on a daily, consistent basis.

• They meet together with Shay, and her mother opens with "Shay, Frank and I don't get a lot of time together. When we are here, one or both of us are doing chores. We're happy to help you with your phone and insurance and continue to pay for the cable. We just feel like you could contribute by helping around the house with regular chores. That way, Dad and I will have time to do some things together that we like to do." Shay's "forgetfulness" is raised as an issue, but Shay says she can manage it, so they agree on an initial trial on the honor system with no reminders.

• Shayleigh agrees to do the grocery shopping and laundry for the family as starters. Her mother figures she can manage the laundry but has doubts about grocery shopping since she hasn't done it. She prepares a detailed list and twice takes Shay shopping with her. She models the first time and observes Shay the second. She does okay with the list, but Mom realizes Shay will need a more specific list for the next independent trip.

• The first week goes fine, but at the end of the second week, Mom and Stepdad are on their last day of clean clothes and the laundry is not done. Midday, Mom texts Shay and makes it clear today is the day. Laundry interferes with Shay's plans that night, and she is aggravated, which she doesn't hide. Her parents are equally aggravated. The next evening they meet with Shay and hammer out an agreement that laundry will always be done by a certain day, and her Mother will text her the day before it is due.

• Two months into this arrangement, her parents are pleased with the progress they and Shay have made. Shay seems pleased and points out after shopping trips that she has become a shrewd bargain hunter and attempts to school her mother in how to be a better shopper.

• Next comes the thornier issue of housecleaning. When the parents bring it up, they get immediate pushback. Shay insists she is doing her part and says they need to carry some of the load. They, in turn, review what they are providing versus her contribution. They give her the option of either housecleaning or working more hours and contributing financially. She says she'll "think it over" but doesn't get back to them about it. When they ask her, she reiterates that it's not fair but doesn't act on either option.

• Having anticipated this possibility, the parents indicate that Shay needs to choose one of the options by the end of the week (2 days hence). If she can't decide, to save money they explain that they are going to drop their expanded cable package and Netflix. Limit setting and follow-through are new experiences for all of them, and Shay decides to wait it out. Her parents drop the cable package and Netflix. Having established some credibility, her mother lets her know that since housecleaning is the issue, their plan is to pay someone to clean the house. To save additional money, she tells Shay that she will need to cover her own phone plan. Shay decides she will pick up at least 10 more work hours per week. They negotiate that she will contribute $50 per week to home expenses and in return they agree to restore the cable service and maintain her phone plan. This covers her monthly phone and half the cable fee, and the parents net an additional $80 per month.

For young adults like James and Shayleigh, who don't have a goal, you need to figure out how they can find a way forward, toward ultimate inde-

> For some young adults, the goal should focus on functioning like a contributing adult.

pendence, and that might mean setting a goal that doesn't have much to do with a particular career path or other long-term outcome, but rather just focusing on functioning more like a self-sufficient, or at least contributing, adult. Shay's parents had an idea for where to start, and they had a reasonable rationale for Shay about why they needed this. In addition, they had anticipated that Shay might have trouble with follow-through and had thought through an approach to address this issue. But, as you will see next with Dylan, the starting point for parents with the young adult is not always evident or easy. For parents with young men or women in this situation, the summary form on pages 144–146 (also available online; see the end of the Contents for information) can get the conversation started and give parents and young adults some different options to consider as a starting point. We have designed this form to elicit tentative commitments from the young adult in various areas (daily living tasks, employment, etc.) while maintaining the young adult's control by offering choices.

Summary Form

Helping Young Adults without a Goal Get Started

NAME: _____

Living Arrangements

1. Where are you currently living?   Home ☐   School ☐   Apartment/house ☐

2. If apartment/house, who is paying the rent?   Split with roommates ☐
   I do alone ☐   I do with help from family ☐

3. If living at home, do you contribute to expenses?   Yes ☐   No ☐
   How much? _____

4. If No, and living at home and working, how much would you agree to contribute to family expenses on a weekly basis? $10 ☐ $20 ☐ $30 ☐   Other amount $ ____

5. If living at home, do you help with daily living tasks?   Yes ☐   No ☐

6. If Yes, which ones: Cooking ☐   Cleaning ☐   Laundry ☐   Yard work ☐
   House repairs ☐   Other: _____

7. If No, check off which two you would agree to doing on a daily or weekly basis, depending on the task? Cooking ☐   Cleaning ☐   Laundry ☐
   Yard work ☐   House repairs ☐   Other _____

Personal Affairs

8. Do you make or manage your own appointments (e.g., medical, dental, employment)? Yes ☐   No ☐

9. If No, who does? _____

10. If No, with help if needed, which ones can you take over in the next 2 months?
    Medical ☐   Dental ☐   Employment ☐   Other:

11. Do you manage your own finances (bank accounts, credit/debit cards, loans, insurance, etc.)? Yes ☐   No ☐

12. If No, who does? _____

13. If No, in the next 2 months which would you like to set up?
    Bank account ☐   Secured credit card ☐   Debit card ☐

14. Do you own your own car? Yes ☐   No ☐

15. If No, how do you get around? _____

(continued)

16. Do you manage your own daily living activities? Shopping ☐   Laundry ☐
    Room cleaning ☐   Other: _____

17. If you do not currently manage all of these activities, which one would you like to
    take over in the next month? Shopping ☐   Laundry ☐   Room cleaning ☐
    Other: _____

18. Do you wake up daily at the same time? Yes ☐   No ☐

19. What time do you usually get up? _____

20. What are your two or three main or preferred activities during the hours you are
    awake? 1. _____   2. _____
    3. _____

21. What do you think you're good at? List up to three talents or skills:
    _____, _____, _____

Highest Education Level

22. GED ☐   High School Diploma ☐   Some College Courses ☐
    Associate's Degree ☐   Bachelor's Degree ☐   Master's Degree ☐   Doctorate ☐

23. What was your high school grade point average? _____

24. Favorite subject? _____ Least favorite? _____

25. What was your college grade point average? _____

26. Area of specialization or major? _____

27. Are you currently attending or planning to return to school in the next 3–6 months?
    Yes ☐   No ☐

28. For what degree or training? _____

29. Do you have or are you currently pursuing any certifications? Yes ☐   No ☐

30. In what area? _____

Employment

31. Are you currently employed? Yes ☐   No ☐

32. What jobs have you held in the past 3 years? For each job, specify part time (pt) or
    full time (ft) _____
    _____
    _____
    _____

(continued)

33. What was your most preferred job? _____
    Least preferred? _____

34. When did you last work? Within the past 3 months ☐   6 months ☐   1 year ☐
    more than a year ☐   never ☐

35. If not currently working, what type of job that you are qualified for would you like
    in the next 3 months? _____

36. If not sure, what employment area would you prefer that you either are qualified for
    or that is entry-level and has minimal qualifications?
    Retail/customer service ☐   Work helping people (e.g., education, health care) ☐
    Information technology ☐
    Physical work (construction, landscaping, custodial, etc) ☐
    Administrative office work ☐   Transportation: driving ☐   Delivery ☐

Executive Skills

37. What are your two or three strongest executive skills?
    1. _____   2. _____
    3. _____

38. What are your three weakest skills? 1. _____
    2. _____   3. _____

Possible Future Goals

39. In the next 5 years, what would you like your job or career to be? _____
    _____

40. In the next 5 years, what would you like your living situation to be?
    Living alone in my own apartment ☐
    Living with roommates in an apartment/house ☐   Living at home ☐
    Other: _____

41. What barriers do you see that could get in the way of your reaching this possible
    goal? _____
    _____
    _____
    _____

42. What types of supports might you need to reach your goal (e.g., additional school
    or training, transportation, living expenses, money for school, tutorial support,
    executive skills support)? _____
    _____
    _____
    _____

Dylan: Stuck at Square One

Dylan isn't working, isn't helping around the house, gets up at his leisure in the morning, and spends his time playing video games and surfing the Internet. In the past, he has taken a few courses at the local community college to see if he could find an area of interest, but nothing really stuck. He's also had a couple of retail jobs in a convenience store and supermarket but was laid off. His parents are at a loss for how to get Dylan interested in becoming independent and asked him to fill out the summary form. His results are shown on pages 148–150.

Next Steps

Setting a goal, particularly one built on reasonable goodness of fit, is cause for celebration because it implies a commitment and underlies motivation. We hope parents and young adults will take a little time to mark this achievement. But as you move forward, please keep in mind a couple of important caveats.

There is a significant gap between goal setting and goal attainment. We opened this chapter by saying that this step is a fulcrum for the entire process of getting a young adult started on independence. Many parents and young adults, however, mistake this pivot point for an endpoint.

Keep in mind that goal setting is the "talk the talk" phase, while goal attainment requires the young adult to "walk the walk." For young adults who are stuck, and particularly for those who evidence executive skills weaknesses, sustaining the effort associated with goal-directed persistence can represent a significant challenge. The neuroscience literature tells us that the energy needed to use a weak executive skill is rapidly depleted. This does not mean that because you have weak executive skill your goal cannot be reached. But it does mean that you will only be able to muster the energy needed to sustain a weak executive skill for short periods of time. If you have set a goal that is 6 months or a year or even more off in the distance, the initial motivation you get from setting that goal will likely not energize you enough to continuously exercise your weak executive skills over that period of time. Instead, the long-term goal needs to be broken down into a series of short-term "mini-goals" that can be accomplished with limited engagement of an executive skill and/or support from others. This means that rather than the long-term time horizon associated with the final goal, we need to rely on shorter-term, brief time horizons associated with each mini-goal. If the time horizon is short, we are much more likely

Sample Summary Form

NAME: _Dylan_

Living Arrangements

1. Where are you currently living? Home ☑ School ☐ Apartment/house ☐

2. If apartment/house, who is paying the rent? Split with roommates ☐
   I do alone ☐   I do with help from family ☐

3. If living at home, do you contribute to expenses? Yes ☐ No ☑
   How much? _____

4. If No, and living at home and working, how much would you agree to contribute to family expenses on a weekly basis? $10 ☑ $20 ☐ $30 ☐ Other amount $ ____

5. If living at home, do you help with daily living tasks? Yes ☐ No ☑

6. If Yes, which ones: Cooking ☐ Cleaning ☐ Laundry ☐ Yard work ☐
   House repairs ☐ Other: _____

7. If No, check off which two you would agree to doing on a daily or weekly basis, depending on the task? Cooking ☑ Cleaning ☐ Laundry ☑
   Yard work ☐ House repairs ☐ Other _____

Personal Affairs

8. Do you make or manage your own appointments (e.g., medical, dental, employment)? Yes ☐ No ☑

9. If No, who does? _Mother_____

10. If No, with help if needed, which ones can you take over in the next 2 months?
    Medical ☑ Dental ☐ Employment ☐ Other:

11. Do you manage your own finances (bank accounts, credit/debit cards, loans, insurance, etc.)? Yes ☐ No ☑

12. If No, who does? _I get money from my parents_____

13. If No, in the next 2 months which would you like to set up?
    Bank account ☐ Secured credit card ☑ Debit card ☐

14. Do you own your own car? Yes ☐ No ☑

15. If No, how do you get around? _Parent's car_____

16. Do you manage your own daily living activities? Shopping ☐ Laundry ☐
    Room cleaning ☑ Other: _____

(continued)

17. If you do not currently manage all of these activities, which one would you like to take over in the next month? Shopping ☐ Laundry ☑ Room cleaning ☐
Other: _____

18. Do you wake up daily at the same time? Yes ☐ No ☑

19. What time do you usually get up? _Between 7 and 11 A.M._____

20. What are your two or three main or preferred activities during the hours you are awake? 1. _Computer games_____ 2. _TV_____
3. _____

21. What do you think you're good at? List up to three talents or skills:
_Computer in general_____, _online gaming_____, _____

Highest Education Level

22. GED ☐ High School Diploma ☑ Some College Courses ☑
Associate's Degree ☐ Bachelor's Degree ☐ Master's Degree ☐ Doctorate ☐

23. What was your high school grade point average? _2.5_____

24. Favorite subject? _Computers, tech ed._____ Least favorite? _History_____

25. What was your college grade point average? _2.2_____

26. Area of specialization or major? _None_____

27. Are you currently attending or planning to return to school in the next 3–6 months?
Yes ☑ No ☐ _Maybe_

28. For what degree or training? _Something with computers_____

29. Do you have or are you currently pursuing any certifications? Yes ☐ No ☑

30. In what area? _____

Employment

31. Are you currently employed? Yes ☐ No ☑

32. What jobs have you held in the past 3 years? For each job, specify part-time (pt) or full time (ft) _Retail, convenience store (pt), supermarket (pt)._____
_____
_____
_____

33. What was your most preferred job? _supermarket cashier_____
Least preferred? _____

(continued)

149

34. When did you last work? Within the past 3 months ☐   6 months ☑   1 year ☐   more than a year ☐   never ☐

35. If not currently working, what type of job that you are qualified for would you like in the next 3 months? _____

36. If not sure, what employment area would you prefer that you either are qualified for or that is entry-level and has minimal qualifications?
    Retail/customer service ☑   Work helping people (e.g., education, health care) ☐
    Information technology ☐
    Physical work (construction, landscaping, custodial, etc) ☑
    Administrative office work ☐   Transportation: driving ☐   Delivery ☐

Executive Skills

37. What are your two or three strongest executive skills?
    1. _Flexibility_   2. _Stress tolerance_
    3. _____

38. What are your three weakest skills? 1. _Goal-directed persistence_
    2. _Task initiation_   3. _Sustained attention unless I like something_

Possible Future Goals

39. In the next 5 years, what would you like your job or career to be? _Something_ _using computers, gaming, or maybe security_

40. In the next 5 years, what would you like your living situation to be?
    Living alone in my own apartment ☐
    Living with roommates in an apartment/house ☑   Living at home ☐
    Other: _____

41. What barriers do you see that could get in the way of your reaching this possible goal? _Money for school subjects I don't like, not enough money to live on my_ _own and get car._
    _____
    _____

42. What types of supports might you need to reach your goal (e.g., additional school or training, transportation, living expenses, money for school, tutorial support, executive skills support)? _Living expenses, money for school_
    _____
    _____
    _____

to be able to maintain the energy needed to exercise our executive skills. In so doing, we achieve two benefits: We improve a weak executive skill through continuous practice, and we accomplish the small, daily steps that build the foundation and stairway to successful long-term goals. The next chapter will show you how to set SMART goals that will help you stay on track.

Success with reaching small initial goals can lead to overconfidence and withdrawal of support and vigilance about the effort needed to keep moving forward. Getting prematurely and excessively confident can interfere with and in some cases derail the goal-attainment process. A series of successes in attaining minigoals naturally builds confidence in the young adult and her parents about the possibility of attaining the "big" goal. On the one hand, that confidence is justified and readily contributes to continued positive momentum. On the other hand, the success can lead to overconfidence about the ease of the journey going forward. Not infrequently, we have encountered parents and young adults who, based on these initial successes, jump to the conclusion that the young adult is "over the hump." The assumption is that obstacles to attaining the goal have been cleared and that the young adult will be able to proceed independently and without the need for additional support. In fact, to pull back on support or to discontinue the vigilance about the effort needed to attain mini-goals often leads to stumbles and falls. The falls, in turn, can significantly undermine the young adult's confidence and the motivation to resume the journey toward the goal. In the remaining chapters in this book we'll try to alert you to places where a plan can fall apart due to overconfidence and lack of vigilance and also give you some strategies for staying on your path.

STEP 6

....

Make It Official
Use SMART Goals to Plan the Steps and Evaluate Progress

If your young adult has completed the summary form in Step 5 and the two of you have agreed that a proposed goal is a good fit, it's time to start the planning phase of this journey to independence. If you're still not convinced that a particular goal is a good fit but the tools you've been using point in that direction, you can start the planning phase anyway. Figuring out how to get to a destination has a way of revealing whether there are so many potholes and roadblocks in the way that it might be a good idea to rethink the ultimate endpoint. So forge ahead; if your young adult needs to come up with a new goal, you have the information and tools to make that turn.

Identifying the Starting Point to Map Out a Rough Timeline

When you think about planning to meet a goal, one of the first factors that comes to mind is time. How long will it take to reach this goal? What's realistic while not being too open ended? The answer to such questions depends a lot on where the starting point is. For young adults like Jonas, who are stymied mainly in finding a career path, the timeline may stretch out over a few years, to allow for occupational research, education/training, and job searches. For young adults like Shayleigh and Dylan, who aren't self-sufficient at all and may be unmotivated to become more independent, the timeline can be quite short. This is in part due to the fact that the goals are likely to be modest (e.g., taking on responsibility for one household chore at a time), although it's also an acknowledgment of low motivation, as discussed below. As you'll see in the rest of this chapter, a longer-term goal will require planning to achieve a few different levels of subgoals. Even a short-term goal, however, should be examined closely for smaller goals that can lead most effectively to the final destination.

Jonas is working and pretty much supporting himself. He needed some encouragement from his mother to get started on a future plan, but with a little nudge from her and some information about himself, he has a potential goal. We know from the summary form that he has a car, helps around the house, and manages his own affairs. Given his school history and executive skills weaknesses, he has some concerns about school. But he's tailored his coursework plan to these concerns, and he's willing to accept some help from his mother, with limits. For him the starting point would seem to be getting specific information about school (courses, schedule, costs, etc.) and choosing a course to start with.

We've also met Cheyenne. She's not quite as far along in the goal-setting department as Jonas. Cheyenne has narrowed her focus to either returning to school and pursuing a marketing major or going in a completely different direction to look at psychological ops and intelligence in the Army. For her, narrowing the choice is a logical next step. This would include getting more detailed information about school and about the Army.

And then consider Dylan, the young man we met for the first time at the end of Step 5. He has a goal (cybersecurity) similar to Jonas's. Given his current baseline, does the same starting point as Jonas, his alter ego above, make sense? Considering what we know about executive skills and what's needed to sustain that effort to meet a goal, we'd venture that it does not. Based on Dylan's current level of self-sufficiency, mustering the effort to get a certificate in cybersecurity will be difficult. At present, he is not managing even the basic daily tasks that reflect self-regulation of behavior.

On the continuum of independence, Dylan is halted at a very early stage of young adult development and shows few signs of either the skill set or the desire to manage his own affairs. His starting point is vastly different from Jonas's, and therefore Dylan's parents can't look at goal setting in the same way as Jonas and his parents. Typically, when we think about the goals of young adults, we think longer-term, toward some type of self-sustaining outcome. While Dylan's parents might hope that cybersecurity represents this outcome, little in his summary supports this view.

If Dylan is to progress toward independence, goals for him need to be concrete, short term, of limited effort, and accomplished in a familiar context. As shown on the goal-setting form Dylan and his parents used (Step 5), the desired outcome is skill building in basic behaviors of independence. Dylan has not shown sustained success outside the home in either school or work, so his goals should be planned in the context of his home environment. One goal component should involve a focus on the activities of daily living that Dylan will need to manage if he is to become self-sufficient. Currently, there is no "cost" to Dylan for the services that he receives at home (meals, Internet access, etc.). Payment should be another goal component and involve work or chores around the house. (Shayleigh's mother and stepfather learned this lesson the hard way when they tried to enforce demands that Shay do chores and errands without imposing a cost—it was when her help around the house became "payment" for her access to the Internet and other provisions from her parents that she became motivated to achieve the goals.) A third goal component involves a new daily routine that will bring Dylan closer to the behaviors he will need to execute if he is to succeed at a job or school, such as a daily schedule of tasks.

If your young adult is stuck at a stage of significant dependence on you, you may be dismayed by the idea that he will have to become proficient in basic self-sufficiency before taking more substantial steps toward independence. However, the advantage in having to start with goals that originate with home and family is that you can provide monitoring and support and have tangible evidence of progress.

Since young adults in this circumstance may show little interest or initiative in formulating these goals, parents can expect to be much more involved in discussion and collaboration about these goals. Pushback by the young adult is not unexpected since change requires effort and can engender anxiety. Parents should be prepared to negotiate with the young adult, exchanging benefits they provide for tasks carried out by the young adult, as Shay's parents did in the previous chapter. See the form on page 155 (also available online; see the end of the Contents for information).

In our discussion of how to get started and maintain momentum, we'll illustrate how the different starting points for Jonas, Cheyenne, and Dylan necessitate different short-term initial goals.

Benefits Provided by Parents to Young Adults

Check off which of the following benefits you are currently providing to your young adult. The purpose of this list is to provide a starting point for the parent(s) and the young adult to collaborate on an agreement about compensation that the young adult can provide to the parents for these benefits. This list is followed by a set of questions regarding what type of contribution, if any, the young adult is currently making to the home and parents. The list is more likely to be applicable if the young adult is living at the home, but parents may be providing some of these benefits to young adults who do not live at home.

Benefits:

☐ Room   ☐ Transportation

☐ Food   ☐ Television

☐ Personal care supplies   ☐ Computer

☐ Prepared meals   ☐ Cell phone

☐ House cleaning   ☐ Cell phone plan

☐ Laundry   ☐ Wi-Fi service

☐ Clothing   ☐ Health insurance

☐ Spending money   ☐ Medical expenses

☐ Other _____

Current or potential contributions by the young adult to compensate for these benefits:

Does the young adult provide any of the following?

☐ Regular payments to you (e.g., from employment)

     If yes, how much weekly? _____

☐ Pay own expenses?   Spending money _____   Transportation _____
     Clothing _____   Personal care items _____   Cell phone plan _____
     Other _____

☐ Consistent help with household chores?   Laundry _____   Dishes _____
     Cleaning _____   Shopping _____   Cooking _____   House repairs _____

☐ Other _____

The Importance of Breaking Down the Goal

Young adults with executive skills weaknesses are likely not just to be stuck right now but also to have a history of unattained goals. Undoubtedly, you've seen the damage these "failures" can do: demoralization, lack of confidence, and more. For parents, it's pretty tough to see your kids feel so bad about themselves. What's important to know at this goal-setting and planning stage is that your son or daughter might resist investing the effort to change his or her behavior in pursuit of a goal and might feel anxious about the potential for another failure. Unfortunately, these two factors can feed on each other: if the young adult chooses to avoid change, he doesn't have to make any effort, and if he makes no effort, he can't possibly fail, which leaves him apparently anxiety free. This outcome is, of course, an illusion. What really happens is that underneath the inertia lies shrinking self-confidence and ballooning anxiety.

The solution? Breaking a goal down into smaller objectives and steps so that each step/task takes little time and requires limited effort. In addition, you have to give the young adult the best chance of succeeding at these small steps, because early success builds behavioral momentum and confidence, establishes realistic expectations, and promotes a working memory of successful problem solving to refer back to. This means the young adult needs to have the skill set to attain the short-term goal and that there are supports in place—transportation, money, and parent(s) readily available to provide emotional and material support for the young adult. We'll have more to say about this and specific strategies to address these potential roadblocks below. The starting point for these strategies is SMART goals.

SMART Goals

SMART goals are the steps that help a person move from a long-term goal that will take a while to complete to the specific action steps that say what the person will do along the way to eventually reach the long-term goal. It's a way to make sure that that plan the person comes up with matches the long-term goal. It also is specific enough so that both the young adult and the parent(s) know whether the young adult is on track to be successful.

For a young adult like Jonas, the long-term goal is to become certified to work in cybersecurity. Obviously, the even longer-term goal is to become employed in cybersecurity, and it could even be to work for a certain company or to attain a particular position. But, as you can see from the definition of

SMART goals below, those goals are a little ill-defined at this time, while certification is not.

It's important to understand that you can attach all different names to different levels of goals. All of the goals should be SMART by our definition. In some configurations, people identify the farthest goal as a "long-term goal" (something that might be a few years off), interim goals as "milestones" (achievements that can be made in a few months to a few years), and the goals that get them to the milestones as the SMART goals, with action steps that get them to each SMART goal, each taking a few days to a week. See the box below.

SEQUENCE OF GOALS

Long-Term Goal

Length: Up to 3 years or longer

A long-term goal is a specific and concrete degree, job, or career that the participant wants to achieve. It should be a good fit for the participant's experiences, skill set, and preferences. For example, Jonas, one of the young adults we've been following, has the long-term goal of working in cybersecurity.

Casey, another of the young adults we've been following, has the long-term goal of becoming an RN.

Milestones

Length: A few months to a few years

Milestones are specific events that signal the accomplishment of significant stages on the journey to the long-term goal, like earning a degree, getting an intermediate job, or completing a training program. For a long-term goal, the young adult may have multiple milestones. Prerequisites can also be milestones for reaching the long-term goal. In his quest, Jonas has four milestones: (1) enrolling in a cybersecurity program, (2) completing semester 1 of program, (3) completing semester 2 of program, (4) applying for cybersecurity jobs.

Casey has four milestones: (1) finding a certified nursing assistant (CNA) job, (2) gaining acceptance into a licensed practical nurse (LPN) program, (3) completing the LPN program and finding a job in the field, (4) and being accepted into an RN program.

SMART Goals

Length: 2 to 4 weeks

SMART goals are needed to reach each milestone: they are specific, mea-surable, attainable, realistic, relevant, and timely. Each participant will have multiple SMART goals. Prerequisites can also be SMART goals in sup-port of the long-term goal. Jonas's first SMART goal is enrollment in a cybersecurity program. Casey's first SMART goal is enrollment in a CNA program.

Action Steps

Length: Up to 1 week

Action steps are the smallest, most immediate steps toward reaching a SMART goal. The participant can make progress with action steps today. Jonas's first action step is identifying available cybersecurity programs. Casey's first action step is identifying available CNA programs.

This entire sequence is spelled out in detail for Jonas below.

For Jonas the long-term goal is to get a job in cybersecurity, milestones include things like completing courses, and SMART goals include tasks like completing courses to obtain the certificate needed for a job in the field. Action steps could include doing most/all the assignments necessary to get agreed-upon grades in the courses. For someone like Dylan or Shayleigh, in contrast, there may not be a clearly articulated long-term goal like a job or a degree or milestones toward reaching it. Rather, there may initially be just SMART goals involving increasing the skills of adult living and contributing to the family's household, like doing household chores. Considering Shay-leigh, for example, a long-term goal, given where she is now, might be consis-tent completion of three household chores and a contribution of $60 weekly for expenses within 5 months. This seems to be a reasonable expectation given where she is currently. The advantage of this goal is that it provides both parents and Shayleigh with a target, and interim steps can be established to evaluate progress.

On page 168 you'll find an example of a SMART goals plan for Jonas, whose long-term goal is to obtain a job in cybersecurity. That plan includes the long-term goal, milestones, SMART goals, and actions steps with deadlines. Jonas's long-term goal will likely involve nearly a year. Casey's, because of how far he needs to go to reach his long-term goal of becoming an RN, could involve 3 or more years.

There are five parts to a SMART goal. Each part corresponds to one of the letters in *SMART*.

- **S *stands for* SPECIFIC.** The SMART goal says exactly what the person wants to happen. It should answer these five W questions:

  - Who is involved? (That's the young adult, so the SMART goal starts with the young adult's words "I will . . . ," then tells what she will do.)

  - What does the young adult want to accomplish? (Get a job? Take a course?)

  - Where will this happen? (At a store? At a hospital? At a community college?)

  - When will it happen by? (Two weeks from today? Before the end of June?)

  - Why is this goal important to me? ("I'll earn more money. I'll be learning something that will help me get the job I want.")

- **M *stands for* MEASURABLE.** If the goal is measurable, it means that the young adult will be able to know for sure when he has reached his goal (The day that I get the job; The day that I get my passing grade back for the course.)

- **A *stands for* ATTAINABLE.** This means that the young adult knows that if she works hard, this is a goal that she knows she can reach by the time she said she will reach it. She either already has the skills and resources that she needs to reach it or can create a plan to get the skills and resources.

- **R *stands for* REALISTIC *and* Relevant.** "My goal is really important to me, so I will make a plan and follow it. I want to reach my goal, and I have the ability to do it."

- **T *stands for* TIMELY.** That means he will reach his goal in a specific amount of time and by a specific date. ("By my birthday, I will save $500.")

SMART goals help the young adult plan a series of specific steps that have short time horizons, which increases the likelihood that they'll be reached. Developing a SMART goal cannot guarantee success, but each element in the SMART goals process allows for an analysis of why any stumble occurred or progress ceased. The following guidelines will help your young adult and you define SMART goals.

GUIDELINES FOR CREATING SMART GOALS

- *The specific goal should begin with the words "I will" followed by a verb or "To" followed by a verb.* For example, "I will contact three employers with job openings that I am qualified for" or "To call three employers who have job openings that I am qualified for." Effective SMART goals avoid opening phrases such as "I want to" or "I'd like to."

- *Each feature of the SMART goal should be written down, and the young adult and the parent should each keep a copy.* We have provided a simple form for that purpose; see the Goal-Setting Worksheet on page 163. Young adults or parents may balk at this step because it seems cumbersome or implies a lack of trust. If either party is uncomfortable with the process, then begin with a verbal commitment to the SMART goal features, and, if necessary, one of you can write them down if recall is an issue. Whether a written record will be necessary going forward will be determined by whether you and your young adult agree, at the deadline, on what you or she committed to to begin with. In some cases, parents may need to develop their own SMART goals because the young adult's attainment of her goal may be contingent on the parent's completing a goal that is a component of this.

- *A date should be attached to each goal.* The young adult has stated what he intends to accomplish, so the next step is to specify by when that will happen. Again, this should be a specific date and, in the interest of keeping the time horizon short, in the relatively near future. We will have more to say about that below.

- *Specificity is an essential part of SMART goals.* "To take some courses" or "to get a job" is too general. To be measurable, the task to be accomplished should be stated in sufficient detail to ensure that the young adult and the parent can agree that the goal has been met. Otherwise, parents and young adults can end up with conflicting expectations. For example, "to get a job" might be satisfied as a goal in the young adult's mind if she finds a job for 10 hours per week. The parent, on the other hand, may have expected that a job meant full-time work. With a goal like "I will find and apply for five full-time jobs in my area of health care within 4 weeks from today," both young adult and parent will be able to determine if the goal has been met.

- *Sharing the goal with someone other than parents can help boost success.* When the young adult shares her goal with close friends on social media, for example, she takes advantage of a technique called "correspondence training." We will have more to say about this in Step 7.

- *Writing down goals and putting them in a place where they can be seen routinely helps goal attainment.* The availability of smart phones and calendars makes it possible to record goals and get regular reminders of what they are.

- *Reviewing and revising goals is inevitable.* For most people, goal setting using this process is a new experience. Success will improve with practice, so it is important not to see goals initially established as set in stone. It will help to review and at times tweak the goals with experience; see page 175.

On pages 162–163 (and also available online; see the end of the Contents for information) you'll find a SMART Goal-Setting Guide, which provides handy reminders of how to formulate SMART goals, and a worksheet for setting goals. Both are useful tools for young adults going through the process of setting up a SMART goal plan.

SMART Goal-Setting Guide and Worksheet

GOAL-SETTING GUIDE

Following are components of an effective goal—one that describes performance standards that will specifically "tell us what effective behavior looks like." The SMART acronym can help us remember these components.

- **S**pecific. The goal should identify a specific action or event that will take place.
- **M**easurable. The goal and its benefits should be quantifiable.
- **A**chievable. The goal should be attainable given available resources.
- **R**ealistic. The goal should require you to stretch some, but allow the likelihood of success.
- **T**imed. The goal should state the time period in which it will be accomplished.

Here are some tips that can help you set effective goals:

1. Develop several goals. A list of two to three items gives you flexibility to work on several things over a period of time.
2. State goals as declarations of intention, rather than items on a wish list. "I want to apply to three schools" conveys a desire but lacks commitment to action. "I will apply to three schools" indicates an intended action.
3. Attach a date to each goal. State what you intend to accomplish and by when. A good list should include some short-term and some long-term goals. You may want two or three goals for 2- or 3-month intervals and four to six for the year.
4. Be specific. "To find a job" is too general; "to find and research five job openings before the end of the month" is specific. Sometimes a vague general goal can be seen as an aspiration, and you can then identify more specific goals to take you there.
5. Share your goals with someone who supports you and cares if you reach them. Sharing your intentions with parents, a sibling, or a best friend will help ensure success.
6. Write down your goals and put them where you will see them or put them in a phone calendar. The more often you read or hear your list, the more skilled and successful you'll become.
7. Review and revise your list. Experiment with different ways of stating your goals. Goal setting improves with practice, so play around with it.

Writing an Effective SMART Goal Statement

Rules for writing goal statements:

1. Use clear, specific language.
2. Start your goal statement with TO + an ACTION VERB.
3. Write your statement using SMART goals criteria.
4. Think positive (avoid negative language)!

(continued)

An example of a goal statement:

To run the mini-marathon this May and complete the 10-mile race in under 1 hour to beat my personal best time.

Notice how the statement above begins with the word "to," includes the action verb "run," and tells "what" (the marathon), "why" (to beat personal best time), and "when" (May).

GOAL-SETTING WORKSHEET

Use the following worksheet to identify the specific **SMART** criteria you will use to write your goal statement.

What is your basic goal? _____

_____

1. Is it **Specific?** (Who? What? Where? When? Why?) _____

_____

2. Is it **Measurable?** How will I measure progress? (How many? How much?) _____

_____

3. Is it **Attainable?** (Can I really do this? Is it attainable with enough effort? What steps are involved?) _____

_____

4. Is it **Realistic?** (What knowledge, skills, and abilities are necessary to reach this goal?)

_____

5. Is it **Time-bound?** (Can I set fixed deadlines? What are the deadlines?) _____

_____

My Goal Statement

Using the guidelines for **SMART** goals writing and your answers to the questions above, write a specific home-, school-, or work-related SMART goal that you would like to achieve in the next 2–3 months. Repeat this exercise as needed to write other SMART goal statements.

_____

_____

_____

Creating a Plan

Now is the time to create a plan for reaching the goal set in Step 5. As we've discussed, the goal can be long or short term or somewhere in between; it can be ambitious or simple. What's important is that the goals and plan be determined by the young adult—with your support and help only—and that they meet the criteria of SMART goals. But because you're likely to be new to this process, we strongly suggest that you consider starting with a relatively short-term goal just to get the hang of the approach. Here are a couple of examples of simple SMART goals:

SMART Goal 1

I will complete my certified nursing course and obtain my certificate by 12/15/18.

Action steps:

1. I will complete my CNA coursework and training by 12/1/18.
2. I will take one CNA practice test every other day for the next week.
3. I will take the CNA test on 12/12/18 at 9:00 A.M.

SMART Goal 2

I will apply for three part-time jobs at businesses near campus within a week.

Action steps (starts on a Tuesday):

1. Go to _____, _____, and _____ to get job applications by Thursday.
2. Complete all three applications by Sunday.
3. Drop off the applications next Monday and ask at each location what the next step is.

Obviously, both of these SMART goals could be included in a longer-term plan for a longer-term goal. If your young adult is like Jonas, who has a long-term goal in mind that fits the criteria for goodness of fit as determined in Step 5, you're probably going to need a more complex plan. We'll show you below how Jonas and his mother sketched out a whole plan for his long-term goal of securing a job in cybersecurity. Meanwhile, take a look at the blank form on page 166, which you can use to create your own plan. It includes lots of space for goals of different levels, and you may not need all of them all at once. We've provided a blank version of the form online (see the end of the Contents for information.)

If you can agree on a simple SMART goal like the two examples above, consider going through the process of entering the goal and action steps in the form. Then you can move on to what is often the trickier part of the process: negotiating time frames.

Negotiating Deadlines for Reaching SMART Goals

If your son or daughter has been stuck for a while, you undoubtedly feel a sense of impatience or even urgency that he or she start reaching goals that will lead to independence, especially if you've reached the stage in your own life when you'd like to enjoy some increased independence or you're concerned about your own resources as retirement looms. This impatience can influence your behavior in collaborating with your young adult, and it's important to stay aware that it might lead you astray in negotiating time frames for goal achievement.

I speak from the experience of having repeatedly had and continuing to have these interactions with Colin. In Step 1, he noted that as the first deadline for this book approached, he felt the undercurrent of almost every interaction with me as the communicative equivalent to the theme to *Jaws*. Since, as of this writing, we still have an arrangement that I will text him when course deadlines approach, he routinely experiences the same undercurrent of Jaws approaching. And ironically, I experience my own sense of anxiety and looming disaster (e.g., failing a course) as deadlines come and go unmet. Interesting that depending on your perspective, the same person can be both predator and prey. Fortunately, Colin mostly tolerates my impatience because we are working under a SMART goals deadline that he set for himself.

Since time frames for accomplishing SMART goals are critical to the success of the young adult moving forward, we will discuss how young adults and parents can negotiate these goals to the satisfaction of both. While the progress of the young adult may never be fast enough for the parent, by accepting the young adult's time frame, the parent reinforces the young adult's autonomy and independence. Jonas offers a good illustration.

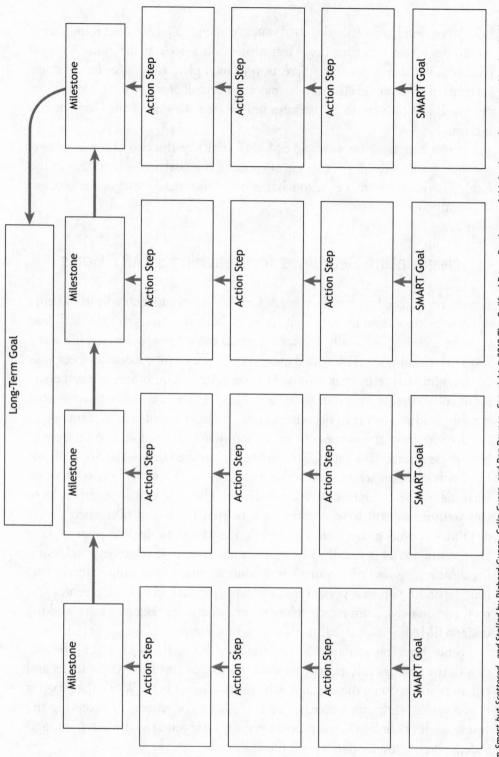

Jonas

On page 168 you'll see the plan Jonas mapped out. Jonas had already determined in Step 5 that his goal of becoming certified in cybersecurity had goodness of fit for him. He has identified the benefit of the goal in that there are jobs available and it is an area that he's interested in. Since he has already taken some college courses and understands what his potential weaknesses are and has chosen an area of interest, he has met the criteria of the goal being specific, measurable, achievable, realistic, and timely. So his long-term goal meets the SMART criteria.

To get an idea of how to reach that goal, Jonas and his mother had to step back from the long-term goal and look at the requirements for certification to work in this area. Jonas established that getting a certificate in cybersecurity will require four courses. Next he had to figure out time frames. Assuming that most community colleges offer 8-week courses, these are the timelines for the longer-term milestones. At the same time, there are potential obstacles to overcome, and so for Jonas and his mother, shorter-term SMART goals will increase the likelihood that he'll keep moving toward the long-term goal. For example, one SMART goal might be to sign up for and complete one cybersecurity course with a grade of B or better within the next 8 weeks.

Jonas now has a reasonable and comparatively short-term first SMART goal, but to ensure that he is in fact on the right path and can overcome potential obstacles, we recommend that he inform his mother of a set of weekly objectives—action steps—that will be accomplished over the period of the 8-week SMART goal. For example, in week 1 he would specifically identify all the requirements and due dates for the first course that he needs to take, as well as access to weekly grade updates. After each course starts, his objective for each week would be on-time and successful completion of the course requirements for the week with objective instructor feedback by the end of the week that he shares with his mother. While this might seem like a high degree of specificity, the objective is to ensure that Jonas can meet the recurring demands of the courses, and weekly monitoring allows for troubleshooting and intervention if he is struggling. For the sake of simplicity, in Jonas's goal chart, we have combined two courses in each SMART goal and 4 weeks in each action step. If we were to spell out the complete chart as described in the text, there would be a SMART goal for each of the four courses and an action step for each of the 8 weeks that a course lasts.

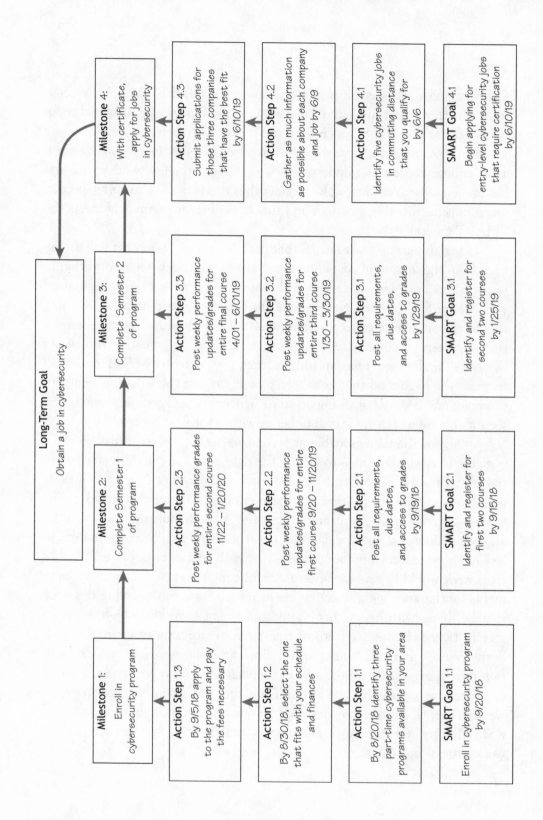

Long-Term Goal

Obtain a job in cybersecurity

Milestone 4:
With certificate, apply for jobs in cybersecurity

Action Step 4.3
Submit applications for those three companies that have the best fit by 6/10/19

Action Step 4.2
Gather as much information as possible about each company and job by 6/9

Action Step 4.1
Identify five cybersecurity jobs in commuting distance that you qualify for by 6/6

SMART Goal 4.1
Begin applying for entry-level cybersecurity jobs that require certification by 6/10/19

Milestone 3:
Complete Semester 2 of program

Action Step 3.3
Post weekly performance updates/grades for entire final course 4/01 – 6/01/19

Action Step 3.2
Post weekly performance updates/grades for entire third course 1/30 – 3/30/19

Action Step 3.1
Post all requirements, due dates, and access to grades by 1/29/19

SMART Goal 3.1
Identify and register for second two courses by 1/25/19

Milestone 2:
Complete Semester 1 of program

Action Step 2.3
Post weekly performance grades for entire second course 11/22 – 1/20/20

Action Step 2.2
Post weekly performance updates/grades for entire first course 9/20 – 11/20/19

Action Step 2.1
Post all requirements, due dates, and access to grades by 9/19/18

SMART Goal 2.1
Identify and register for first two courses by 9/15/18

Milestone 1:
Enroll in cybersecurity program

Action Step 1.3
By 9/15/18 apply to the program and pay the fees necessary

Action Step 1.2
By 8/30/18, select the one that fits with your schedule and finances

Action Step 1.1
By 8/20/18 identify three part-time cybersecurity programs available in your area

SMART Goal 1.1
Enroll in cybersecurity program by 9/20/18

Cheyenne

Cheyenne is in a different place in terms of the goal-setting process. Her use of SMART goals shows that this process can be used even before a final longer-term goal is set. With her dad's help she's come up with two potential goals that are viable, but she needs to know more about what it would take to reach the goals before she can say that they're probably a good fit for her. Whereas Jonas had already looked into the first steps he would need to take to get into cyber-security, including certificate courses and programs, Cheyenne needs to gather more preliminary information about the marketing and armed services options before committing to either. Cheyenne is excited about some possibilities she can sink her teeth into. For her, a SMART goal involving information gathering would help move the process along toward a good-fit goal. In addition, with concrete information in hand, she would already have a start on next steps when she makes a choice.

Cheyenne's SMART goal then could be the following: By 4 weeks from today, I will have contacted and met with Army, Navy, and Air Force recruiters regarding my interest in intelligence and psychological operations. As part of that goal, by the end of this week, I will have gotten specific information online about the qualifications that I need to enlist, the type of commitment I would need to make, and the potential benefits to me. I will also obtain online information from my previous college about the requirements for a marketing major, what I need to do for readmission to school, and what current tuition is.

These relatively short-term goals meet the SMART criteria and put Cheyenne in a good position to decide whether she meets the goodness of fit criteria and remains interested in the armed services or marketing as goals. If so, with the information she has gathered, Cheyenne will be able to determine next steps.

Dylan

For Dylan and his parents, there are quite different options. One is to accept him at his word—that is, he really wants to obtain a certificate in cybersecurity as an entry card to this field. This can constitute a long-term goal and, with answers to a few questions (number of courses needed, time frame, etc.), could lead to a legitimate set of short-term SMART goals and related action steps. At the same time, his history and current behaviors make it a stretch to frame this as a good-fit goal for Dylan. His interest in computers is confined to online games and Internet information of high interest. His academic history is limited and shaky, and he currently evidences few of the behaviors needed to participate actively in college coursework and assignments. In addition, he has no financial resources to contribute.

Why would a parent sign on to this or a similar situation? Because we want to help and support our children. And because for many parents, hope springs eternal. If your young adult is dead in the water, so to speak, any proposed goal that moves the process forward and isn't completely unrealistic may seem worth the risk. If you and your young adult want to try, there are easy ways to minimize the risk by using the SMART goal approach in a compressed time frame. For example, Dylan could say, "Within 2 weeks, I will identify three colleges with online cybersecurity certificate programs, identify the number of courses each one requires, and determine the least expensive of the programs. I will also identify the type of experience necessary for an entry-level job in cybersecurity, the number of jobs currently available within a 30-mile radius, and the typical starting salary range of those jobs." This short-term SMART goal seems well within his skill set since he can accomplish it at his computer and at his leisure. His action plan for achieving this SMART goal would look like this:

Steps to Follow to Complete Goal	Target Completion Date	#1 Not Done	#2 Done
1. Contact three colleges with online programs and get number of courses needed by each for certificate and costs of each college.	7/19		
2. Search Internet for type of experience necessary for entry-level cybersecurity job.	7/22		
3. Identify entry-level cybersecurity jobs and starting salaries within 30 miles of my home.	7/25		

Young adults who are in Dylan's position and need to start small can use the form on page 171 (also available online; see the end of the Contents for information) instead of the more complex form Jonas used. With the online form you can add or subtract cells to the form to accommodate more or fewer steps toward the goal. Note that the form allows young adults to review how they did on reaching the goal and what the next step is—revising the goal if things did not go well or setting a new SMART goal if the first one was attained.

Suppose Dylan doesn't meet this short-term SMART goal, that is, doesn't even get the initial information regarding courses or jobs. What should be the

Action Plan for Achieving a Short-Term SMART Goal

Steps to Follow to Complete Goal	Target Completion Date	#1 Not Done	#2 Done

Did you follow the plan?

What worked well?

What didn't work so well?

Next step: ☐ Revise plan   ☐ Make new SMART goal and action plan next step for him and his parents? The next step *should not* be a continuation of the same goal or allowing more time to meet it. Why? For Dylan, cybersecurity was a questionable goal to begin with, given his history and current starting point. The short-term goal above was a reasonable starting point, was well within his wheelhouse, and required minimal effort using a skill set he already possesses. As such, this was an assessment of his readiness for change, his motivation. He did not pass the test. Hence, for now, the cybersecurity goal should be set aside, perhaps to be revisited later.

> *When a young adult fails to meet a short-term goal even though the goal was a good fit, readiness for change or motivation is usually lacking and the goal needs to be set aside for now.*

If Dylan does meet the short-term goal and obtains the necessary, preliminary information about cybersecurity, as a sign of good faith, his parents could support his taking one course and building goals around this course (e.g., on-time completion of assignments, certain grade performance). This would minimize their risk while at the same time letting Dylan build some sense of success and confidence.

For Dylan and his parents, there is both an upside and a downside to this course of action. And interestingly, they share the same features. The upside is that Dylan can maintain his current lifestyle, including his daily routine (get up when he wants, play games on his computer, etc.). This increases the likelihood of success since he will be operating well within his current skill set and habits. The downside is that Dylan has little "skin in the game." That is, he doesn't have to make any change in his current habits and has no financial stake.

There are other issues. Dylan's academic history does not suggest a strong track record of commitment to college. Nonetheless, for now let's give him the benefit of the doubt. If he is able to attain a certificate, the next real challenge will be a job. Dylan lacks a recent employment history of any type. And he has a well-habituated daily lifestyle (e.g., wake when he wants, dress as he wants, and do what he wants) that clashes with the expectations of a consistent, daily work environment. These include following an employer's decisions about time of arrival, hours, dress, and execution of the job requirements.

Daily Living and Work Goals

What, then, should be the next steps for Dylan and his parents? Interestingly, regardless of whether he has or hasn't met the short-term goal of information gathering, the next steps are similar. Assuming he hasn't met the short-term goal, school is off the table for now as a goal. SMART goals should then be in the two areas that will most quickly increase Dylan's independence and self-sufficiency: daily living skills in the form of chores around the home and a job. The type of chores that he starts with can be negotiated with his parents. If he is willing, morning chores, particularly when his parents are still home, have the dual advantage of establishing a regular wake-up time (which he may need for work) and having parents around to prompt him. For example, he might make the coffee, get his own breakfast, and put the breakfast dishes in the dishwasher. This could become the following SMART goal: On Mondays, Wednesdays, and Fridays for the next 3 weeks, Dylan will make the morning coffee, get his own breakfast, and clear the family breakfast dishes. If, instead, Dylan wants to choose his own chore(s), they should meet at least the three-times-a-week criterion, make an observable difference in the environment, relieve the parents of something they currently do, and be completed before they arrive home from work. For example, Shayleigh's parents, after a less than successful first attempt, collaborated on a plan with her that was satisfactory to all and resulted in Shayleigh's increased self-sufficiency.

A SMART short-term work goal for Dylan might be the following: "By the end of this week, Friday, I will identify two different types of entry-level jobs (e.g., retail sales, manual labor) that I would be willing to do. I will identify and save on my computer a total of at least five job openings in one or both areas, any type of experience required, and the application process. By the end of next week, Friday, I will have submitted applications for at least three of those jobs. I will only consider jobs that can offer 20 or more hours per week."

Suppose, on the other hand, that Dylan both met the short-term goal and started the coursework. Would that materially alter the approach above, which is focused on daily living and work goals? We think not, for the following reasons. Dylan's history and current baseline or starting behaviors suggest that, even should he finish school, transition to work may be difficult. Other than having a certificate in hand, we can imagine that 10 months hence, his situation might not be significantly different. Independent living and work require that he develop and practice skills like planning and prioritization, time management, response inhibition, and task initiation, among others. Can he formulate a plan for his day, get himself up in the morning, initiate and sustain attention to tasks such as chores and work that are effortful and not preferred? Can he inhibit the temptation to stay in bed or play video games? These behaviors are unlikely in the absence of consistent practice in daily living and work situations. So to beef up his chances of success in more independent living and making use of his potential certificate, we'd suggest the same course of action as above with one minor modification. In searching for a job, any type of work related to computers would be an advantage. That said, however, Dylan is not in a position to be picky, and work experience in any job trumps continued unemployment.

Next Steps toward Implementation of Goals

If your young adult identified a long-term goal with goodness of fit in Step 5, and you've collaboratively set SMART goals that meet the criteria discussed in this chapter and identify specific short-term tasks that, strung together, will lead to the long-term goal, you've completed the "talk the talk" phase. (You're at the same point even if all you've decided to work on right now is a simple short-term goal so the young adult can make progress in skills of independent functioning at home and in the work world.) Now you're ready to begin the "walk the walk" phase, the real acid test for the path to goal achievement.

Reviewing and Clarifying SMART Goals

A critical part of this phase is evaluating whether goals are being met as laid out in the action plans written. A tool that you'll find useful for this job is the form on page 175 (also available online; see the end of the Contents for information), which allows you to (1) evaluate whether, from your perspective, a specific SMART goal set by the young adult has been met and (2) determine what aspect of the goal was not met and why. (*Please keep in mind that this tool is not intended for use as a critique of the young adult's performance or as a means for you to decide what you think is a better SMART goal for the young adult.*)

With this information in hand, you can discuss your thoughts with the young adult to get her perspective and to collaborate on what additional clarification in the SMART goals criteria would help going forward.

Let's face it, most if not all of us have had the experience of committing to a goal and then losing momentum or getting sidetracked. If you and your young adult have followed the plans we've suggested so far, you've built a foundation for success. But what if the process is interrupted? What if Jonas doesn't complete his coursework on time? Or if Cheyenne doesn't call a recruiter? Or if Dylan gets distracted during the chore he committed to? These stumbles and stalls do not represent failure. They simply point to a need to review and revise.

A lot of different factors could be playing a role. Is there any mismatch between the skills and characteristics of the young adult and the SMART goal?

Evaluating Success with Achieving SMART Goals

What was your young adult's SMART goal? _____

From your perspective, was the goal met? Yes, completely ☐   Yes, partially ☐
Not at all ☐

If you believe the goal was not met, from your perspective, what would help going forward? _____

1. Was it **Specific?** (Who? What? Where? When? Why?) Yes ☐   No ☐

   Do you think it was too vague? If so, what might be added? _____

   _____

2. Was it **Measurable?** How was progress measured? (How many? How much?)

   How many or how much was going to be attained? Was a more specific number needed? _____

   _____

3. Was it **Attainable?** Could this realistically be attained? (With enough effort? What steps were involved?) Would more support have helped? _____

   Was the goal attained? Completely ☐   Partially ☐   Not at all ☐

4. Was it **Realistic?** (What knowledge, skills, and abilities were necessary to reach this goal?) _____

   _____

   _____

   Did the young adult have the knowledge, skills, or abilities to attain the goal? Would more experience or support help the young adult? _____

   _____

   _____

5. Was it **Time-bound**? (Were there fixed deadlines? What were the deadlines?) _____

   _____

   _____

   Were the deadlines met? Completely ☐   Partially ☐   Not at all ☐

If, for some reason, there *is* a mismatch between the skills of the young adult and the task demands of the SMART goal, progress will come to a halt. How do we determine the presence of a mismatch? The most basic source of a mismatch involves a skill deficit in the young adult directly related to the task. For example, the young adult doesn't know the procedure for washing clothes, or making medical appointments, or preparing a meal. If your young adult's starting point is daily living activities, unless you have observed him or her performing the task independently at some point, don't assume he or she has the skill. You can do a walk-through of the task with him or her, or, if that is too intrusive, have him or her describe the steps of the task or provide a list of task steps.

If the young adult has the basic skills, a second problem source might be the design of the SMART goal. If parents and young adults disagree about whether the goal was met, the issue often involves the goal not being specific enough or lacking clear measurement criteria. Beyond that, was the goal realistic and attainable, given the young adult's starting point? Or was the timeline too short? In our experience, such issues arise when parents explicitly pressure young adults to reach for more than they are ready for or when young adults take on the extra reach because they want to meet parental expectations.

For the young adults addressed in this book, if they have the basic skills and SMART goals are well designed, a mismatch is most likely the result of a discrepancy between executive skills and task demands. Let's say Jonas has started his first course in the cybersecurity sequence. He successfully completes the week 1 assignments on time but misses the week 2 deadline for posting a short paper. He started it but got distracted playing "Call of Duty" online with friends. In and of itself, you might think this is no big deal. We see it differently. The missed deadline reflects Jonas's weaknesses in the executive skills of sustained attention and time management. And his past failure to manage college was in good part due precisely to these kinds of issues. Okay, suppose we have identified a situation where Jonas's weak executive skills clash with the task demands of school and cause a halt in his progress. What do we recommend that Jonas and/or his mother do about it? How do we resolve task/executive skills mismatches? We've identified three major intervention strategies to improve goodness of fit between executive skills and task demands: *modifying the environment, using a motivator, and strengthening the executive skills.* In the next chapter, we'll examine each of these in detail and offer specific strategies and examples.

STEP 7

....

Make It Easier
Anticipate Problems and Intervene
to Get Things Done

For young adults with executive skills weaknesses, the likelihood of a stumble or stall on the way to their goal is quite high. The best way to minimize the negative consequences is obviously to anticipate and plan for the stumbles. In this step you and your young adult have an opportunity to think about the young adult's particular executive skills weaknesses—as well as your own since this will be important information to factor into how you can and can't help—and how the young adult can get around them, while tackling upcoming action steps to reach the SMART goals identified in Step 6. Before you start working on that, however, we want to repeat an important caveat: Remember that control belongs to the young adult here, as it has throughout the first six steps of this journey.

How to Support the Young Adult in Meeting Challenges on the Way to Goal Achievement

1. *View any stumble by the young adult as just that—a stumble, like falling off the bike used to be.* The only appropriate conclusion to draw about this stumble is that it indicates the plan didn't work as it was set up and needs to be tweaked.

Let's go back to Jonas for a minute. He missed a deadline as a result of weak time awareness and distractibility. Suppose Jonas and his mother talk and, based on the discussion, he makes two changes. He sets a sequence of alarm reminders

177

on his phone and works in a location where he doesn't have a Wi-Fi connection. As a result, he completes the task on time. In this case, he's recognized his executive skills weaknesses and modified his environment (alarm, location change) to compensate for these weaknesses. Whereas initially, under the original task conditions, he couldn't succeed, now he can. His mother approached this stumble as a task–skill mismatch and discussed with Jonas how to address it.

But what if his mother forgot everything she's learned about collaboration and thought, "He just doesn't want to do it—it's just like the last time he was in school; nothing's changed"? Seeing the behavior of the young adult as evidence of a refusal to change or lack of effort ends the collaboration and leads to nothing but confrontation, blame, and an attempt to coerce or force the change. Think about it: If you were trying to lose weight, get organized, or save money (New Year's resolution, anyone?), and you had a setback and heard "You're just lazy" from those who knew about your goal, would you be motivated to keep trying? Or would you be more inspired by hearing "What can I do to help or support you?" or "I'm behind you all the way; stick with it!"? You know the drill. The challenge is to follow it: do your best to suppress any accusations of character flaws or lack of effort when your young adult stumbles and keep offering open-ended support.

2. *The young adult must be the person who chooses what, if any, strategy to use to address a weak area.* Colin and I can personally attest to this being a delicate topic. When a stumble occurs, parents can provide material and emotional supports as stepping stones on the young adult's path. They can model, suggest, and assist with the implementation of strategies to facilitate problem solutions. And, in some cases, they can "nudge" the young adult to adopt one or another of the problem-solving strategies below by appealing to the young adult's sense of fairness, desire for independence. or some reward or "payoff." Or the parent can nudge the young adult by making continued support contingent on some objective measure of increased self-sufficiency. However, the parent *cannot, indeed must not,* insist that the young adult choose any particular strategy.

If the young adult doesn't or can't settle on an effective intervention to move the process along, parents can (1) offer the young adult a reward to motivate and jump-start the process and/or (2) gradually reduce support if there is no visible progress toward self-sufficiency. We prefer the first option since it feels less coercive and is less likely to provoke conflict. Consider adding the second element only if option 1 doesn't work to your reasonable satisfaction.

3. *If you want to present problem-solving approaches, watch out for coercion.* Young adults who are reading this book along with you will be able to read about the strategies we suggest and can choose them on their own. In fact, it's wise to read through the strategies before launching the plan you two agreed on in Step 6. Getting a preview may help the young adult know exactly what to do when a stumble occurs, or she may want to put some of the tools in place before beginning to work on an action step.

BEFORE WORKING ON THE FIRST ACTION STEP, ASK YOURSELVES:

- What might be a stumbling block for me in accomplishing this step?
- What problems have I had with tasks like this?
- What, if any, strategies or tools have helped me get around this challenge?

Then, as you read through the strategies in the three tables in this chapter, take note of the ones that immediately seem like they might be of help in completing this first action step. Repeat with subsequent action steps.

If you're reading the book on your own, the most direct way to suggest solutions is to give the young adult a copy of the strategies to read. You could say something like this: "Hey, Col, you've said that getting started on the papers for your courses [i.e., task initiation] has been an issue. I got these out of this book and have been able to use them for myself. They're not a miracle solution, but they might be of some help." A second option, if you're pretty familiar with your young adult's roadblocks, is to talk about a few different options that are tailored to the roadblock. With Colin, for example, when he's in his own apartment, surrounded by his sources of distraction (computer, phone, TV, etc.), getting started or maintaining focus has been an issue, so sometimes he comes to our house to work. A third option, if you share a weakness with your young adult, is to model the strategy and comment on its effectiveness. For example, if I'm having trouble getting some writing finished, I ask my colleague Peg to give me a deadline. Colin has seen me do this, and we've talked about it. Recently, when I've asked him about writing I need from him, he either asks me for or gives me a specific time by which it will be completed and usually meets or even beats his deadline.

*   *   *

The bottom line in supporting rather than controlling management of challenges is to use this approach: If the young adult wants initially to be off on her own without parental assistance of any kind, then in the interest of independence and autonomy, she should do that. You can introduce the strategies as potential problem-solving tools and the young adult can choose or not choose to use them. That said, if you're providing some type of support (spending money, rent assistance, room and board, tuition, etc.), it is reasonable to negotiate with the young adult about next steps if the goal is not met and hasn't been met in the time frame initially specified. We'll have more to say about this in the scenario commentaries below.

At this step you'll learn three different ways to tackle potential or actual problems in task completion and goal achievement caused by executive skills weaknesses: environmental modifications, ways to enhance motivation, and direct improvement of executive skills.

Environmental Modifications for Executive Skills Weaknesses

The place to start in grappling with executive skills weaknesses is to look for ways to *work around them.* This can be done by modifying your environment either to support your weak executive skills or to reduce the negative impact of that weak skill. Note that we're using the term "environment" in the broadest sense. Young adults who bump up against a problem that arises from a weak executive skill should start by asking three questions:

1. *Can I alter the physical or social environment in which the problem arises to lessen the problem?*

2. *Can I modify the task I'm trying to accomplish so that it demands less of my weak skill?*

3. *Is there some way I can recruit people around me (friends, family, coworkers) to help me manage my weak skill more effectively?*

We recommend turning to environmental modifications first because these types of interventions are the quickest and easiest to implement and we're big believers in avoiding unnecessary effort. Also, once you've found an effective set of environmental modifications for a particular executive skills weakness, they can become part of a toolbox you can use whenever that weakness rears its head.

In the descriptions that follow, you'll notice that the three domains of environmental modifications often overlap, but it's helpful to identify the categories because this classification can act as a cue or mnemonic device as you think about how to make adjustments for your weak executive skills.

Offloading

One way in which the environmental modifications overlap is that many of them take advantage of a process that the brain science literature calls "offloading." Offloading refers to giving over some of our cognitive functions to technology, which in this context means any tool outside of ourselves that relieves us of having to carry a certain mental function, such as remembering information, within our own brains. For example, at its simplest level, a list can be a piece of cognitive technology. Rather than carrying within our own working memory the food you need to buy, you can offload this information by writing a grocery list. Then you need only to remember to take the list with you and look at it when you arrive at the supermarket.

Of course, young adults (and some parents) are highly familiar with much more sophisticated technology for offloading. Smart phones and their apps offer a virtually limitless supply of tools that allow us to offload information and plans. (You'll read about a number of them in action from Colin in Step 8.) This technology also supplies us with the means to activate our attention to particular situations or events. We have cars that prompt our attention when we've drifted into a lane of passing or oncoming traffic. We have cars that alert us to approaching cars when we are about to back up. And now we have cars that, should we forget to brake in time, activate braking systems for us. When we alphabetize books on our bookshelf or practice putting our keys and cell phones in a particular location we've used the principle of offloading even though no technology in the sense we usually use the term is involved.

> *Offloading, a strategy we all use in daily life, can be a boon to young adults with executive skills weaknesses.*

So a fourth question to ask yourself:

4. *Is there some way I can offload aspects of the task that make it effortful and therefore likely to be avoided?*

Modifying the Physical or Social Environment

Picture your living spaces—each room in your house, what your car looks like, the inside of your refrigerator—and ask yourself, "If I change some part of these physical spaces, would my executive skills weakness be less of an impediment?" Or look at your social world and see if there are conflicts and tensions inherent in that world that are likely to bring your executive skills weaknesses to the fore. Can you redesign your physical environment or change your social environment to improve the situation?

Table 1 (below) lists each of the executive skills and provides an example of how the physical or social environment might be altered to make the executive skills weakness less of an intrusion.

TABLE 1. ALTERING THE PHYSICAL OR SOCIAL ENVIRONMENT

Executive skills weakness	Examples of modification to physical or social environment. If this executive skill is a weakness for you, you might:
Response inhibition	First, identify the impulsive behavior that gets you in trouble (e.g., spending/drinking too much at bars, making comments on social media sites). Avoiding the situation is one option. Another is short-circuiting the behavior. For the bar, leave credit cards at home and limit the amount of money you take. For social media, write down in advance what you won't say.
Working memory	If you leave home without things, the low-tech option is to put things near the door so you see or trip over them. On your cell phone, the *tileapp.com* is worth looking at. You attach small tiles to keys, etc., and use your phone to activate an alarm or, if you lose your phone, you can press a tile to locate it. If you forget appointments, when you set them up immediately put them on a calendar.
	It's a bit more involved, but you can make access to a preferred object contingent on remembering something. For example, lock a preferred item in a container at work and tape a key to the container under the light switch or thermostat at home.
Emotional control	If a person or situation pushes your buttons, write down why you interact with the person or put yourself in the situation and decide if you can avoid it. If not, or if there is some positive part of the situation, make rules for what you will or will not talk about. I (Colin) can get pretty hot about politics, so I avoid talking politics at work.
	When a situation comes up unexpectedly and you feel anxiety or anger, use the feeling as a prompt to count to 10.

(continued)

Executive skills weakness	Examples of modification to physical or social environment. If this executive skill is a weakness for you, you might:
Flexibility	Ask people, in advance of an event, what is going to happen in as much detail as possible. Let people know in advance what your plans are and tell them that you struggle when there are unexpected changes in plans. Ask people to surprise you with unexpected, positive events, like taking you out for coffee or lunch.
	In a group of friends or coworkers, let them choose things like where to eat or shop and what time to meet. This will build flexibility and allows you some choice over the situations in which you use it.
Task initiation	Make the task seem less overwhelming by deciding in advance one small part to work on or a small amount of time (e.g., 5–10 minutes) to work on it. In the early stages, stick to the limit you set. (This also can be considered a task modification.)
	"I won't lie down on the bed till I put away laundry." "I will open the school website as soon as I go on the computer."
Sustained attention	Distractions are the enemy of sustained attention. Identify your most tempting distractions and cut off your access to them by shutting them off, making them hard to get to by putting them in another location, or by moving yourself to a different location where they are unavailable.
	"If I spend 60 seconds on this computer screen (timed), I can have a mini-M&M."
Organization	Start small by picking one thing (dirty laundry, dishes), a consistent place where you'll put these things (laundry basket, sink), and a designated time and amount of time that you'll spend picking up (e.g., just before bed for 5 minutes max). Add another thing only when the first task has become a routine. (Thus, over time, this becomes a habit or skill.)
Planning/ prioritization	Put a large whiteboard on your wall, get a daily calendar, make a to-do list for a set part of the day (e.g., morning, evening). Make a short list (three to five activities max) that you want to do for the day (e.g., work out, do laundry, watch favorite TV show). If it's a project (e.g., clean the bathroom), write the project title at the top to remind you, and list the steps needed to complete the project.
	Pick a goal for yourself for the fun of it and plan it out.

(continued)

Executive skills weakness	Examples of modification to physical or social environment. If this executive skill is a weakness for you, you might:
Time management/ estimation Time urgency/ deadlines	Set all your clocks (and your watch) ahead by 5–10 minutes to give yourself an extra time cushion to get ready for something. Schedule three events in a day planner or on a whiteboard, write down the start time, and estimate the completion time. When the task is done, write the actual time it took. Set a series of alarms that mark the beginning point of the task and when it must be done. Put time in between everything you do as a buffer. Add at least 20% more time to every estimate you make.
Goal-directed persistence	Use an auditory or visual prompt daily to ask what you did to further your goal for the day and put a notation (one or two words) of anything you did on a calendar. Get inspirational quotes about achieving goals and use a different quote each day, setting it on a random schedule as a reminder on your phone or computer. Post-its work for some people but they have to be in a place where you can't ignore them (on your car's rearview mirror, in the middle of your computer screen). Set aside a small amount of money daily to buy something you want in 2 weeks.
Metacognition	Identify two characteristics that enable you to perform well in your work or home environment and then list two that get in the way of doing those jobs. Post them in that setting to remind you to use your strengths and not let your weaknesses interfere. As in the modification above, the post has to be in a place where you can't ignore it. Take a task or situation you were successful at and write down the steps you did to make it successful.
Stress tolerance	Think about ways to make your environment feel less stressful—preferred music, reduced clutter, quieter. Take a break away from the situation and do an activity that needs some of your attention but is not too challenging, like an easy video game, puzzle, or sorting activity like laundry. Get to work early before your coworkers so you can spend more of your working hours in a reduced-stress environment. Imagine a stressful situation you've been in and see yourself getting through it by using a specific coping strategy like muscle relaxation.

Adapted from *The Smart but Scattered Guide to Success* by Peg Dawson and Richard Guare (2016).

Modifying the Task

Task modifications are designed to help people cope more successfully with the fallout from a weakness in an executive skill the task requires. That's why the strategies in Table 2 (below) are not broken down by executive skill: these strategies are not aimed at improving the executive skill itself, and many task modifications in fact work across skills.

> Task initiation and time management have always been bugaboos of mine. Even when I'm able to start a large project, I frequently get bogged down in aspects that are trivial. As a solution, I often now tell my dad or girlfriend that I will e-mail a certain quantity per unit of time (e.g., a page of an essay per 90 minutes). There is no other component, but having the work broken down piecemeal and tied to someone I feel accountable to helps me get started and be economical with my time. I can even conduct a sort of performance review afterward, since the pace and quality of my work is preserved in the e-mails.

TABLE 2. WAYS TO MODIFY TASKS

Task modification	Explanation
Make the task shorter or build in breaks.	A key reason we avoid effortful tasks is that we think *they will take forever!* Ask yourself how much time are you able to tolerate on the unpleasant task and then either spend only that amount of time per day or divide the task into small, manageable portions by building in breaks.
Use a 1–10 scale to find ways to make the task feel less effortful.	Ask yourself how effortful the task feels on a scale from 1 (it's a snap, requires no effort, and you may actually enjoy doing it) to 10 (you hate it and will put it off as long as possible). Then ask yourself how can you turn the 8–9–10 task into a 2–3–4 task (it's unlikely you can turn a 10 task into a 1, so don't even try). For example, is there a way to make it shorter, easier, put it on someone else's chore list, pay someone to do it? Some of the other suggestions in this table may give you additional ideas for how to do this.
Pair the unpleasant task with something pleasant.	Examples: listen to music or books on tape while exercising; watch a movie while sorting laundry; find someone to do the task with you—or to keep you company while you do it.

(continued)

Task modification	Explanation
Do the unpleasant task or use it as a "filler" when engaged in another activity that has a more automatic component to it so that you can "kill two birds with one stone."	Do the task while riding on a bus, train, or in a car or at the laundromat.
Give yourself something to look forward to doing when the effortful task is done.	With children, we use the refrain *First work, then play*. The same principle can work with adults. Complete three job applications, then spend 15 minutes on a social media site (set a timer!). Pick one task on your to-do list, complete it, and play a video game.
Break the task into very small pieces, make a written checklist with each piece, and make a first–then bargain with yourself after you check off each three pieces.	If necessary, include a column that reads "start time" and build in a reminder such as a smart phone alarm to help you remember to start the task.
Use technology such as tablets and smart phones to build in cues and reminders.	Calendars on the computer or smart phone can be programmed to remind you of an obligation at set times (e.g., 24 hours before, 10 minutes before); reminder programs can not only be used to create to-do lists but can also be programmed to cue you to complete the item either at a specific time or at a specific location (e.g., when you walk in the door to your house after work). Post-it programs are useful, too—especially if you program them to appear on your desktop as soon as you turn on your computer. (Don't have too many, and if the reminder doesn't get you to do it, dump it!).
Turn open-ended tasks into closed-ended tasks.	Artificially make a task closed-ended by time, amount, or meeting one criterion. For example, convert "clean up the kitchen" to "put the dirty dishes and forks, etc., in the dishwasher, napkins in the laundry, and wipe the table." If you're not sure how to do this, enlist the help of someone else to do this with/for you.
Build in variety or choice. (Remember that novelty is reinforcing and helps you to sustain attention.)	Sometimes what makes things feel like drudgery is the sheer unchanging routine of it all. Think about ways to "mix it up" with respect to effortful chores. Could you change the *order* in which you do a set of tasks, or could you do them a different way, could you build in surprise (e.g., put each task on a separate slip of paper and put them all in a jar; do the first one you pull out—and add in some fun things to do too so there's always a chance that the next slip you draw out won't be work at all!)?

Adapted from *The Smart but Scattered Guide to Success* by Peg Dawson and Richard Guare (2016).

Getting Others to Help

For this type of environmental modification we're addressing young adults directly, because it's particularly important for the independence seeker to take the lead here. Soliciting help with executive skills challenges might be considered just another way to engineer your social environment to support weak executive skills, but we think it merits its own category because some of the options can be pretty powerful. They also come with the potential for misuse, which we'll spell out as we go along.

There are ways that your family, friends, and coworkers can provide supports to help you work around or compensate for weak executive skills (there are also things they can do to support your efforts to *improve* your executive skills, but that will be taken up later in the chapter).

It makes sense to ask for help that taps another person's executive skills strengths (check the results from the Relationships-Based Executive Skills Questionnaire in Step 4 if you need a reminder), but keep in mind that your requests need to be reasonable. If you're asking your parent, he or she is not likely to feel imposed on. But if you're asking a coworker or friend, it's important to be mindful of imposing without offering something in return. If your weakness involves a task that other people are depending on you for, asking them to understand or compensate for your weaknesses (repeatedly) without making an effort to improve is not likely to be well received. For example, if you're a member of a team that has a production quota and you're not contributing your fair share because you have an executive skill weakness, team members may appreciate and even empathize with you. But at the end of the day, understanding and empathy will wear thin if the team loses a bonus, for example, because you didn't deliver.

We have indicated throughout these steps that as a rule it's the young adult rather than the parent who needs to set the standard for progress or improvement of performance. But we recognize that there can be exceptions to the young adult as the sole decision maker. For example, if the parent has a significant stake in what the young adult is doing, such as paying for tuition, it is reasonable

> *When asking others for help, show that you're making efforts to improve so you may not always need the same help in areas of weakness.*

for the parent to have some say. Our caveat is that parents must guard against making unrealistic demands, such as in the case of school (e.g., dean's list every semester, attendance only at certain schools, or insistence on a specific type of degree). While the parent may see these demands as "getting my money's worth," such demands are in fact coercive. On the other hand, expecting adequate levels of performance such as "C's or better" is reasonable. If the young adult balks at this, the best option, in the case of school, is that he take out loans. Parents have the option of helping with repayment if the young adult has shown reasonable progress.

Table 3 on page 189 identifies ways you can recruit people around you to help you manage your weak executive skills. If the parent is the source of executive skills support, we recommend a "Let me tell/teach you how to best help me" approach in which the young adult takes the lead in deciding how the parent can help and determine what specific help will be needed. This also includes, from the young adult, "what not to say/do and a way for me to let you know that you need to stop" (e.g., by using a single gesture, word). It's very easy, when your adult child is stuck, to slip back into the parent role of "Take my advice, I know from experience," which gets back to coercion rather than collaboration.

Identifying and Using a Reward as a Motivator

In Step 2, we explained that motivation is an essential component of readiness for change. We also said the best foundation for motivation is for the young adult to identify a desired goal. But for long-term goals the promise of a distant achievement is rarely enough to keep the young adult on track. For many people, a short-term reward provides the little push they need. If you're trying to get in shape by going to the gym every morning before work, but on some days you wake up to pouring rain or frigid outdoor temperatures, you might not be moved to head out just by thinking of the ultimate endpoint of getting in shape. Maybe the short-term reward you need is buying new athletic shoes or clothes, or posting on Facebook that you met your goal for the day, or having coffee with your friend after you're done, or a phone upgrade. Using weak executive skills, which are needed to reach a goal, requires significant effort, and the energy needed to exert that effort is rapidly depleted. Having a short-term reward to look forward to helps *energize* a person to persist through the effort.

For young adults with long-term goals, the end goal is but a distant speck on the time horizon that can be reached only by completing a lengthy series of effortful daily tasks that challenge their executive skills. And successful completion of 1 day's or even 1 week's tasks, in comparison to the total distance that needs to be traveled, doesn't even appear to move the needle. Think about Jonas, for example. His four-course cybersecurity sequence may involve 80 or more assignments. Does Jonas's completion of one assignment make him feel

TABLE 3. LOOKING TO OTHERS TO HELP YOU MANAGE YOUR EXECUTIVE SKILLS WEAKNESSES

What others can do	Explanation
Agree to cue or remind you.	If you know you will have trouble remembering something, it may help if you ask someone with a good working memory to remind you. This is particularly helpful when working memory or task initiation is the weak area. But it can also be useful at other times—for example, if you have trouble reading people and you miss cues that you're talking too much or too loudly (i.e., weak metacognition). Having a friend who can give you a little sign when it's time to stop talking can be helpful.
Hold you accountable for your commitments—or just be there to accept your verbal promises.	Research shows that if you make a public commitment to doing something, you're more likely to do it. It's called *correspondence training*. Often, the act of making the commitment alone increases the likelihood that you will engage in the behavior you promised to do—but if that's not enough, a gentle reminder may do the trick. When we discuss skills on page 192, we'll tell you about another set of techniques that are a related but powerful addition to correspondence training.
Provide encouragement and positive feedback. You can also do this this via self-praise statements and self-recording of specific progress you've made on a task or problem.	Research shows that a ratio of three positives for every piece of corrective feedback can change behavior all by itself. We give this advice to parents for shaping behavior in their children, but as an adult, you may have to solicit positive feedback from others. Be honest: tell them, "This is hard for me and I'm working on it. If you notice me actually pulling it off—or even coming close—could you give me some positive feedback about that? It might really help."
Enlist the help of a person who is strong in an area you struggle with. (This is Dick—I mentioned earlier that in conflicts with my daughter, emotional control can be my weakness. Colin is a much more reasoned voice in these situations, so I ask for his help when I'm stuck.) Parents need to keep this in mind because it helps to build a foundation of mutual assistance between you and your young adult.	Look at your executive skills strengths and weaknesses and see how they make some tasks easier to do than others. Then identify the strengths and weaknesses of others that you work (or live) with. Suggest a trade—you'll do something that's easy for you but hard for your parent, friend, or coworker if he or she might help you in a situation that you struggle with and they have a strength in.

Adapted from *The Smart but Scattered Guide to Success* by Peg Dawson and Richard Guare (2016).

like the end is in sight? Especially in light of the fact that these tasks tax his executive skills and he has appealing and more immediately available distractions? In our experience, that's very unlikely.

Think of the long-term goal as trying to reach the top of a long flight of stairs. When the end is barely in sight, one step closer seems insignificant. In part, SMART goals address this issue since they are shorter-term, more immediate goals. SMART goals are like a short (e.g., four stairs) flight with the landing representing completion of the SMART goal. Each flight is a benchmark toward the big goal, but for the young adult the end (landing) is in sight and hence seems more doable. When executive skills come into play, as they do for Jonas with weak task initiation and sustained attention, even each step, such as the on-time completion of one assignment, can be an issue. So the rewards or incentives need to be broken down so that at the end of this one task there is a small payoff.

Boosting Energy and Motivation to Sustain Effort

Russell Barkley notes in his 2012 book *Executive Functions* that certain more immediate incentives can replenish energy needed to maintain effort and help maintain motivation. These include:

- Visualizing the good outcomes/rewards as a result of successful execution
- Using self-efficacy statements before and during task
- Generating positive emotions
- Getting periodic, small rewards throughout the executive skills task

We might not initially think of them as rewards or incentives, but in fact they can be quite powerful, particularly when a young adult can incorporate and use them regularly over time.

Visualizing Positive Outcomes

Visualizing outcomes as a result of successful execution capitalizes on why we are actually engaging in the task. Each individual step represents completion of an action step needed to reach that SMART goal. If Jonas's first SMART goal is the successful completion of the first course in his cybersecurity sequence, and it's an 8-week course, there are eight steps for Jonas to reach the SMART goal. Each time Jonas began working on that week's assignments, he could visualize successfully completing each step and achieving a good grade in the course. If he wants to take this visualization a little further, he can create a graphic for himself, seeing that he has completed, say, 20% of his journey toward his certificate.

We know from motivational research that evaluating your own progress can also be a powerful motivator, so we recommend that the young adult keep a graphic representation of successful achievement of each step using a visual of her choice. This could include coloring in or checking off blocks on a chart or steps on a flight of stairs. There are also a number of different tracking apps that allow us to keep continuous information about our progress.

Self-Efficacy Statements

The value of talking to yourself about what you will do and/or when you will do it and then commenting on performance during the task is well known in sports psychology. For the young adult, a self-efficacy statement might be "I'm going to start this task in 10 minutes and work on it, with one 5-minute break, for half an hour." During the task the young adult might say to himself, "I started on time and I'm making good progress toward completion."

Generating Positive Emotions

Positive emotions can be generated by the young adult and also by those around her. We generate our own positive emotions and increase self-confidence in our ability when we state ahead of time what we'll do to complete the task successfully or overcome a stumbling block and then again when we make positive self-statements afterward. Acknowledgment of success by other people (family, friends, coworkers) can also be a source of positive emotions, particularly if the praise and recognition is focused on the effort that we made to solve the problem. Recognition of effort by other people, even if the outcome hasn't met our expectations, has the effect of encouraging continued attempts to engage in problem solving. To the extent that you and others are working directly with a young adult on her goals, your acknowledgment of her efforts will encourage persistence.

Periodic Small Rewards

Having a preferred activity or object to look forward to after completing effortful work can have a particularly powerful impact on task initiation, sustained attention during the task, and persistence in task completion. Small rewards are most effective when they are determined by the young adult and selected from his repertoire of preferred activities or objects. We've found the most effective way to arrange them is on the basis of the "first–then" schedule, so that getting to the preferred activity or object is dependent on first completing the effortful work. Jonas might say to himself, for example, "As soon as I finish and post the course assignment for this week, I can join my friends in an online game." These types of "first–then" schedules are most effective when they are designed by the young adult since she will be most familiar with her preferred activities and can arrange the schedule in such a way that some or all of a particular piece of work is the criterion for engaging in the desirable activity.

We've now provided two of three key components for addressing specific executive skills weaknesses and the role they can play in the young adult's stall on the path to independence. Thus, the toolbox of intervention strategies available for young adults and parents is nearly complete. The third component involves strategies to directly address the manifestation of the executive skills weaknesses and can incorporate environmental modifications and rewards as well as skill-building strategies.

Improving Executive Skills

When we talk about directly improving executive skills, we need to be clear about what we mean. The objective is to improve the executive skills *behaviors* that get in the way of the specific goal you want to accomplish. If you work on the behaviors most likely to get in the way of your goal, you'll be able to strengthen that skill and use it each time you run into the roadblock. Consider Colin, for example. His long-term goal was to get his BA degree. To do that he needed to complete weekly assignments in a satisfactory, timely fashion, which required task initiation and time management, two of his weak skills. For Colin, these skill weaknesses occurred in the context of school tasks that he found tedious and time-consuming but did not occur in other situations. For example, he didn't have trouble making fantasy football draft deadlines or getting to work on time and carrying out his responsibilities there. So when we talk about improving executive skills, we need to focus on executive skills behaviors in the specific situations or contexts that block the path to our goal, usually situations that are mentally or physically effortful for us.

> *Directly improving executive skills means improving executive skills* behaviors *that stand in the way of reaching your goal.*

To improve executive skills behaviors, the first task in this process is identifying your executive skills strengths and weaknesses, which you did in Step 1. Next comes identifying the specific activities or situations in which your weaknesses occur. With this information in hand, you're ready to address the executive skills behaviors that are obstacles to your long-term goal.

Correspondence Training: Making Yourself Accountable

When we make a firm decision to change a behavior to achieve a goal, we often refer to this as a resolution (think New Year's): "I want this, and I will do this to accomplish it." In our past work we have relied on an intervention strategy called "correspondence training" to help people achieve goals. Correspondence training is grounded in the evidence-based concept that making a verbal or written commitment to engage in a specific behavior at a specific time in a specific context increases the likelihood that the person will carry out the behavior. We mentioned this strategy in Table 3. In essence it involves a way of making yourself accountable to someone by announcing your intention. This could range from Jonas's making a verbal commitment to his mom to work on course assignments for 90 minutes (12–1:30 P.M.) every Saturday and Sunday and submitting complete assignments on time during each 8-week cybersecurity course to his announcing the same intention on social media and asking a friend to check in with him each Sunday about whether he's fulfilling his resolution. Colin did this and gave me access to his weekly assignment posts as added determination for himself. Cheyenne could tell her best friend that she is interested in joining the military and in the next 10 days she is going to meet with Army, Navy, and Air Force recruiters to find out the qualifications for a career in military intelligence. At the end of the 10 days she might arrange to have lunch with her friend to update her. Knowing that you've made a public commitment has incentive value of its own; face-to-face contact with those who know what you said you wanted to do adds to the motivation to follow through on resolutions.

Newer Strategies for Strengthening Resolutions to Change

While correspondence training has been a reasonably effective approach, in the past 5–10 years we have observed the emergence of a set of newer evidence-based strategies that relate directly to people's strong resolutions to change their behavior to meet a goal. We believe these techniques represent a more detailed and effective set of strategies for achieving improvement in executive skills and behavior change. There are three components to these techniques:

- The first, *implementation intention,* is defined as a plan, framed in an *if–then* contingency, that specifies precisely what behavior you will do, in a specific situation, at a specific time. For example, for someone who is trying to lose weight, "At the _____ restaurant tonight, after the meal is over and, if the dessert cart comes out, I will immediately look away and order a cappuccino."

- The second, *mental contrasting,* is designed to complement and increase the likelihood of completing an implementation intention. The technique involves two components. The first involves thinking about your goal, seeing yourself achieve it, and visualizing the specific positive aspects and the good feelings you will experience. The second component involves now thinking about obstacles that could get, or in fact have gotten, in your way of achieving the goal in the past. This is followed by visualizing a behavior that you've decided on to overcome the obstacle and using it successfully.

- The third, *mental simulation,* involves a combination of the first two techniques. You see yourself entering the situation in all the specifics you've chosen above and figuratively walking through the entire situation. You see all the details of the context and see yourself implementing the intentions, imagining the good outcome, encountering the anticipated obstacles, and overcoming them to achieve the desired result and the payoff.

Jonas, for example, would see himself at noon on Sunday, just getting ready to start an online test when a friend texts to go surfing. Jonas would see himself reading the text, texting back that he is tied up until 2:00 P.M., and then see himself completing the test, getting a B+, and proudly telling his mom. Cheyenne would envision herself getting ready to go to the Army recruiter's office later today with a list of questions she and her dad have discussed that she wants to ask. She then visualizes her friend calling that morning and suggesting that maybe Cheyenne should take more time to think about the service instead of meeting with the recruiter. Cheyenne sees herself telling her friend that she appreciates her concern but really wants to get some information. She thanks her friend for her thoughts and tells her she will call her when she gets back. She then sees herself talking with the recruiter, getting more information than she expected, and feeling proud of herself about taking this first step.

In using these techniques, you prepare yourself for the next time you'll be in the situation in which you want to change the outcome. Because you've developed and practiced a detailed visualization, when you're present in the situation, the details have a strong probability of eliciting the strategies and behaviors that you mentally rehearsed. As just noted, these techniques offer young adults the option of using environmental modifications, rewards, and self-generated thoughts and behaviors alone or in any combination. The young adult is encouraged to use whatever seems most likely to lead to successfully addressing the problem and moving on.

Troubleshooting for Missed Steps

The following issues or impediments are among the most common that we see when young adults and parents are working on the development of executive skills. Building these skills requires a combination of one or another of the strategies we've discussed plus regular practice. The bulleted items below represent typical missing elements in improvement plans and quick remedies for them. **Remember, the practice of any executive skill starts with initiation of a behavior related to that skill in the context or situation where you have struggled with that behavior.** Impediments and solutions to these task or behavioral initiations include the following:

- Lack of a specific plan or specific schedule
   Solution: Implementation intentions with mental contrasting and mental simulations: "I *will* begin this task/behavior in this setting [specify both] at this time [specify hour and A.M., P.M.]," publicly stated to family member, friend, or socially media contact, and preferably in writing.

- Lack of a specific, timely, and recurring prompt
   Solution: Auditory and/or visual signal provided by smart phone, tablet, computer, or person via app, social media, phone call/text, in person.

- Lack of a specific, valuable first–then contingency
   Solution: Implementations intentions with mental contrasting and mental simulations: "*First* I will start/finish [specify task] and *then* I will do/watch/go to [specify activity that you value and look forward to].

- Presence and easy availability of attractive distractions such as a smart phone, computer, TV, friends
   Solution: Remove distractions or change environments so that distractions are temporarily unavailable until the *first* part of the *first–then* contingency is complete.

- Lack of energy

   Solution: Modify the task so that it is shorter or requires less effort. Make the payoff in the first–then contingency something that is highly valued.

- Presence of stress

   Solution: Use positive self-statements and brief relaxation strategies; enlist assistance such as support and encouragement from friends or family via face-to-face, phone, text, or social media communications. Modify the task so that it is shorter or requires less effort. Make the payoff in the first–then contingency something that is highly valued.

In Step 8, we give you the opportunity to dig more deeply into all of these strategies and see how they can be applied in real-life situations that typically bring up problems related to specific executive skills. These scenarios will feel very familiar to many readers because they come from real experience: these are Colin's stories, written from his own experiences and those of young adults he has helped to coach and has met over the years on his own journey. In Step 9, we take a short detour to offer strategies if you've come to a roadblock and feel stuck. In Step 10, we show you how the young adults we've been following through this book pulled everything together and learned to build on their own success so that your young adult can do the same.

STEP 8

....

Get Creative to Tackle
Specific Weaknesses

In Step 7 you were introduced to an array of strategies the young adult (with parental or other help as requested) can use to overcome executive skills challenges in working through the action steps that lead to achieving SMART goals. Many of you may feel comfortable running with those ideas and could skip this step if the strategies have quickly become part of your collaborative repertoire. You can always come back to this chapter if you need a nudge that will help you apply the strategies more effectively down the road. For others, integrating the Step 7 strategies into work on action steps may feel more foreign. In that case, this step can kickstart progress for both young adults and parents. Young adults, you'll get a closer look at how to parse problems that may be very familiar to you. Seeing how others experience the same executive skills challenges and then reading a list of practical solutions can help you see where you could apply these tools to your own tasks. Parents, you'll get a look into your young adult's head and what it really feels like moment to moment to struggle with particular executive skills weaknesses. For both of you, these stories are intended to boost empathy and collaboration and inspire creativity.

These vignettes are based on Colin's experiences in his own life and in the lives of other young adults he has observed. In choosing these particular vignettes we have tried to highlight the typical issues that arise for young adults when a skill is weak, many of which come up in the pursuit of independence, from job hunting and job success to renting an apartment and other requirements of self-sufficiency.

After each scenario that follows, we'll note what we've found to be the best categories of solutions and then give some particulars. The best solutions will almost always involve a combination of environmental modifications and skill building through cognitive practice, but the order in which you apply them varies depending on the skill addressed, as do other factors. Before you decide to adopt the solutions we present to the challenges described, we strongly encourage you to practice using the implementation intentions, mental contrasting, and mental simulation techniques on some simple problem areas you want to tackle. This practice significantly increases the likelihood of success.

> **Response Inhibition**—The capacity to think before you act; this ability to resist the urge to say or do something allows us the time to evaluate a situation and how our behavior might impact it.

Mike sat down hard on the couch in his parents' living room, resting his elbows on his knees and rubbing his temples. He fished his phone out of his pocket and logged into his banking app. He glanced at his phone, then quickly punched the home key and looked around the room. Val walked in.

"I put the stuff from the pockets of your laundry in a plastic bag by the door. Can you take care of that in the near future? When you leave the bag on the ground, the dog eats it. You know him: anything with an interesting smell is worth at least tasting."

"Yeah, sure, Mom—sorry, no problem." Mike breathed a temporary sigh of relief, but her having not seen his restaurant and bar tabs didn't pay them either. His checking balance was $180 below what it had been yesterday.

("Why do you do this? Nobody else does. Nobody else 'feels obligated,' nobody thinks you have money to burn, nobody thinks much of it, and nobody remembers 'the gesture' except you!") Mike rubbed right below his eyes and began to plan. He planned for possibilities—that he would need gas money, need a way to prolong paying his student loans, car payment, prolong repaying his parents the money he had borrowed to go to a bachelor party in Atlantic City. Something would need to be stretched out, and Mike thought with increasing anxiety which one would be the easiest to draw out and cause the least distress to the party on the other side. It never got easier, and Mike started to wonder how people can stop themselves from doing something they never think about in the first place.

This particular brand of response inhibition is one that parents think will solve itself when their kid is spending his or her own money. Maybe; maybe with a very high cost; maybe not. We only need to look at historical rates of credit card debt to know that young adults aren't the only ones who take financial leaps without looking. Of course, responsible adults are often in significant credit card debt for legitimate reasons, but for many people the debt is fueled by "want" rather than "need." Spending money fast and hard, and regretting it later, befalls most of us at one time or another. As always, this is about a difference of degree and frequency.

In Mike's case, putting the important but tangential possibility of alcohol intoxication aside (I used this example because of its ubiquity; shopping could also work; any sort of reckless spending is the target behavior), the best remedy, one that quite a few people employ, is to severely limit your access to money prior to going out. As we suggested in Table 1 on pages 182–184, leave your credit or debit cards at home and take only cash. Have your paychecks direct-deposited into a separate branch savings account with no ATM card. While there are reasons that going out on the town with only limited cash might not be feasible, you can create personal barriers that can be broken down in event of an emergency but still present sufficient difficulty to deter irrational sprees.

> *The best solutions?* Environmental modifications, then skill building. In the early stages of trying to manage or improve response inhibition when the temptation is right in front of the person, not giving in is quite effortful. So "out of sight, out of mind" is the way to go. There are a few variations:

• Eliminate the temptation from the environment. This can be effective for a young adult who is routinely in the environment, for example, apartment or home. If other people live there, their cooperation is needed. This can work well for items like junk food and alcohol. It can also work for tempting events like video games if the absence of game controls is sufficient. If you find you're still likely to buy the tempting object, it can be helpful to enlist help from a friend or family member.

• You also can eliminate the means to respond to the temptation; take along limited cash and no ATM or credit card, as in Mike's case. If need be, ask a friend you go out with who has good response inhibition to prompt you.

• Over time you can build response inhibition, or "willpower," using the cognitive techniques of implementation intentions and mental simulation rehearsals as long as you start with low-level temptations and gradually increase the demand.

• You can also build the skill of delayed gratification by saving money for an object or activity in the future and graphing your progress. It's best to start with shorter time horizons so the goal seems in sight.

> **Working Memory**—The ability to hold information in memory while performing complex tasks; it incorporates the ability to draw on past learning or experience to apply to the situation at hand or to project into the future.

6:30 A.M. *Wake up, walk to shower, stop to look at clean laundry basket for options, continue walking to shower.*

6:32. *Shower, wash,* (mental note) *buy more suction cup hooks for loofahs: buy soap; water pressure lower than desired; minor scum around drain—girlfriend will likely not notice; low priority; grab A & L wedding card/project binder/Mom's EZpass before leaving. Okay, now scratch scum with toenail, pick scum out of toenail, soap toe, rinse . . .*

6:48. *Drying off. Need to shave, razor dead battery; don't need to shave, plug in razor.* (Remember) *wallet on dresser . . .*

6:51. *Picking clothes from laundry basket, pick shirt, pick underwear, pick shorts, pick new shirt, pick socks. Go to phone on dresser, turn off snooze alarm, open dresser, pick new shorts, find belt, check phone, no texts, close phone. Home tonight? Not sure, take phone charger from wall, check phone, put phone and charger in pocket. Desired shoes in room? Not sure, put on other shoes.*

7:09. *Desired departure 7:45. Check phone, look through texts, one text from Sandra—work re: morning meeting, necessary departure now 7:30, open fridge, scan, remove yogurt and cold chicken, begin to eat, check phone, no more texts, scan room once more for desired shoes.*

7:25. *Pick another new shirt, check phone, one new text, Sandra: plz bring project binder,* (Remember) *grab project binder . . .*

7:29. *Brush teeth, test razor for juice, sufficient power, shave quickly, razor dead halfway through, buy new razor* (Remember), *keys, go downstairs, get chicken from counter, see desired shoes, change shoes.*

7:35. *Leave apartment.*

7:36. *Return to apartment, grab keys* (mental note), *clean before girlfriend arrival (drain?) . . . leave.*

This is an abridged version of a morning I think most people have had at some point. By abridged, I mean that a real-time incident like this for me would run several pages and include dozens of notes, some of which I probably create in my head and forget so fast I'm barely aware they occurred.

There is an issue of sustained attention here also, reflected in rapid jumps from one focal point to another. This compounds the working memory problem by multiplying elements to remember. Our thinker does exhibit some ability to prioritize on the fly, but not enough to moderate the thought flow.

> *The best solutions?* Environmental modifications first, followed by skill building. Given both the volume and the diversity of items to be remembered, the question is how? A few solutions present themselves.

• The first and probably most important is the use of offloading strategies that involve organization of the physical environment and events. For any object that is used routinely, such as clothing for the morning, selecting the items and putting them in the same location nightly reduces working memory demands. This also holds true for keys, phones, backpacks, as well as personal care items such as razors and toiletries. For events, schedules and shopping lists with audio prompts can be offloaded to smart phones.

• A second skill activity is prioritizing the tasks to be remembered. People usually prefer setting priorities according to personal importance. A list by time (near term to later term) is a related strategy, but importance gives you the option of dropping less important, near-term tasks if pressed for time. Personal planning and prioritizing enhance offloading strategies since they then reflect what is most important.

• While offloading and organization are always helpful, the reality is that physical and digital spaces cannot manage all responsibilities in advance. So an ability to retain information in the short term will always be a necessity. To develop this skill, cognitive or mental rehearsal, seeing oneself in a specific situation carrying out a series of actions, increases the likelihood of success when the real actions are needed. Routinely practicing this type of rehearsal enhances working memory.

> **Emotional Control**—The ability to manage emotions in order to achieve goals, complete tasks, or control and direct behavior.

"Hello, Morton residence, Mr. Morton speaking."

(Mock serious tone) *"Hello, Mr. Morton, this is your daughter, Cassie, er Cassandra Morton calling. Dad, come on, when you answer the phone it's like calling the governor's mansion, lighten up.*

"Cass, I've told you, telephone etiquette is important, which you'd do well to remember."

"Yeah, okay, Dad, whatever. Is Mom there? I've got some news for her."

"Not presently; she had some errands and will be out until later this afternoon. But you can tell me, and I can give her the information when she arrives."

(Short hesitation) Ahh . . . , it's okay, I can wait till she's there."

"Cass, is this bad news?"

"No, no, Dad, not at all. In fact, it's good news!"

"Well, in that case, let me in on your news."

(Hesitation) "Okay, but promise me you'll hear me out completely before you say anything at all."

"Cass, is this really necessary?"

"Please, Dad, just promise."

"All right, I promise."

(Excited) "I, well we, found a place to live, a house, on the bus route so I can get into work at the registrar's office and not have to take my car and hunt or pay for parking! Three bedrooms, one and a half baths, $1,600 a month plus about $200 for utilities . . ."

"Cass, who's the . . . ?"

"Dad, stop! I need to finish! $600 a month each and there's a laundromat around the corner. Other people are interested, so we gave the guy a $300 deposit to hold it. We need the last month's rent plus an $800 damage deposit. LaDana and DJ and I will split the $2,400 for this. I don't have the cash right now, but if you'll . . . we can work out a repayment. Isn't it great!? And like you and Mom have wanted, you can have your place back and I can be out of your hair! What do you think?"

(Long pause) "Cass, I don't think it's a good idea. It's not cheap, and I can't support having a male roommate."

"Well, big surprise, right? I have a great plan to move forward and it doesn't meet your standard? I knew it—same crap, different day, never quite good enough! You know what? I don't give a damn what you think! I'm doing it."

"If you do this, you do it without my financial support, so good luck."

"Screw your support, your Victorian morals, and your precious financial support! I don't need it, and whatever I have to do will be worth it so I don't have to be around you anymore!"

"That's quite enough, Cass! Call when you change your mind and your tone."

"Hell will freeze over first!"

This is the classic case of the inflexibility of the father meeting the weak emotional control of the daughter. Based on her past experience, Cass came tantalizingly close to avoiding this by deferring the conversation till her mother was available. She tried to minimize the risk by extracting her father's promise to listen, but it wasn't enough, and his reaction to her proposed change triggered her reaction to reject his opinion. Once the explosion occurred, their positions became polarized, and resolution through negotiation unlikely. For Cass, she tried the best option, starting with her mother, who likely has played the role of intermediary in the past. Her mother remains her best option, but the interchange has made her mother's work more complicated.

> **The best solutions?** Skill building plus environmental modifications. In the case of weak emotional control, effective management of one's reaction begins well before entering a situation of potential conflict.

• The first skill-building step is to develop an awareness of your hot button issues. That also means the executive skill of metacognition needs to be at least average. If it's a significant weakness, you'll need to ask a family member, friend, or colleague to help you identify your behavioral triggers. Knowing these, if it's an option, change the environment and avoid the topic or situation (e.g., Colin's example earlier of no politics at work). This is not an option when the hot button is a person, such as a parent, manager, or team member you must interact with. In this case, the best option is using an intermediary like the other parent or a sibling (My daughter calls her brother, Colin, to intervene with me.)

• If appropriate, ask someone who can help prompt or mediate your reaction to accompany you to the meeting.

• If the topic involves information the person will react to, sending it in an e-mail or text can pave the way, especially if the information involves other people who can be copied.

• But if none of these are options and you must talk to the person, practice the situation in your head before you see (or call) the person, even to the point of scripting what you'll say. For a work situation, ask a trusted coworker who knows the person to help coach you in your practice. As part of this rehearsal, develop an exit strategy to use if you start to get upset so you don't explode or overreact.

> **Task Initiation**—The ability to begin projects or tasks, without procras-
> tination, in an efficient and timely fashion. Reflects how hard it is to get
> started on a task or situation that you know needs to be completed, in
> spite of the fact that delays will come back to bite you later.

VON: *Ya, you got the Sunday scaries, Sarah. Sunday scaries is that feeling
when the weekend's over, Monday's coming, you got stuff due, but you
try to ignore it, you just sit there.*

SARAH: *(Laughs.) Yeah, thanks, Von.*

*Sarah thinks . . . Von's right, Sunday scaries. Four in the afternoon, at
my keyboard for almost 6 hours, and I'v done nothing on the problem set.
I've been on Facebook, Snapchat, watched TV, started a load of laundry.
I don't know why this happens, but I've got to get past it—it's making me
crazy.*

*So, okay, 4:00 now, and the problems are due at midnight. Eight
hours, enough time, plenty of time really. Even at one set an hour, that's
only 4 hours. And they won't take that long; the professor wouldn't have
them take that long. So 4 hours. So let me get away from this for a second.
I'll go away from this for a second and come back at 5:00, start at 5:00 and
be done by 9:00. If I eat dinner, then by 9:30. So I'll do what I want for an
hour, and then I'll get going.*

So in this Attack of the Sunday Scaries, I see a couple of red flags right
away. First, Sarah's making important but uninformed judgments about the
time she'll need and then letting them percolate into her plan till they become
an assumed fact: 1 hour per set. Second, she seems to be engaging in planning,
goal setting, and time management, but mistakes planning for execution. At
the end of this plan, Sarah seems positive and resolved about doing the work,
but she fails to capitalize on that momentum and instead gives herself the first
hour free. The plan is a false flag of initiation; I've done it many times. Often,
for me, moments like Sarah's come as a crescendo of stress on Sundays, resulting
in delaying some dreaded task. And rationalizing the delay with a shiny new
plan is very gratifying to someone who feels anxious and guilty. For those of us
who struggle with task initiation, plans that start with a break are plans that
can't be trusted.

> **The best solutions?** Environmental modification followed by skill build-
> ing.

• Since effective procrastination involves distractions to occupy attention and avoid the task, a change of location where the usual distractions are not available can be a good first step. The next step is to build a little momentum. We often avoid tasks because they seem so overwhelming. A much smaller task-time commitment can reduce the effortfulness of starting (I'll work on it for 10 minutes). The other option to build momentum is to start doing some other task that requires some effort, but not as much as the one you are avoiding, and gradually working toward the more effortful task.

• Start with the simplest fix, a straightforward change of scenery. Take your computer to a public place where other people are working, to a room with no TV, to your parents' kitchen, to the laundromat where you're killing two birds with one stone.

• Another technique I (Colin) like is a sort of "Dante's Inferno of tasks." Doing effortful tasks builds task initiation. If I'm avoiding a task, I will start doing a less unpleasant but not enjoyable task, like washing dishes or answering e-mails. Then I move to something more difficult or that I like less. I always, ALWAYS, make sure these tasks are of a fixed quantity or length of time, and preferably short, under an hour or even 20–30 minutes at a pop. As I move farther down the list, that thing I'm avoiding starts to look relatively less unpleasant than whatever I'm doing. At that moment, I turn to that task and give it a go, with the caveat that I can return to my list if I choose to do so at the end of a fixed amount of time. And I use a timer on my phone whenever possible.

• For people with weak task initiation, eliminating the source of procrastination is a key environmental modification, hence the benefit of location change. If there are prompts, like people working, in the place you move to that reinforce on-task behavior, all the better. Since daydreaming can be an internal source of procrastination, an external prompt such as an intermittent auditory beep paired with a self-talk strategy ("Stay on task'") on a smart phone can bring you back from your reverie.

> **Sustained Attention**—The capacity to maintain attention to a situation or task in spite of distractibility, fatigue, or boredom.

"Hey, Joe, how goes the job? Any questions or anything I can help with?"

"Hey, Donyelle, thanks for asking, I guess it's going okay . . . well . . . Nah, never mind. I'm sure I'll figure it out."

"Joe, listen, it's a lot to get used to, and at first it feels really fast. My first week, I felt like totally lost and I was sure I'd get fired. Jimbo was my training coordinator, and he saved my butt—let me know that getting this stuff down is tough at first. Now I'm him, so what's up?"

"Working drive-through, I don't know. I've screwed up a couple orders already, and people get pissed. My last job didn't work out 'cause of this, and I need the money."

"Yeah, I saw it on your job app, but your rep is also 'hard worker,' so they'll cut you some slack."

"You think?"

"Most def. Just need to sort this piece out."

"I'm trying to really pay attention, but when it's busy I get stressed and screw up."

"Hey, it happens, so here's something a couple of us did, actually still do sometimes. When you ask and then get the order and put it in the computer, before you process it, read it back to the customer and ask if you got it right."

"Geez, that'll take forever. Won't people get pissed at that?"

"Uh-uh, takes only a few seconds and nobody has complained, I think because they think it's good customer service."

On the face of it, Joe's difficulty might seem like one of working memory rather than or in addition to attention. In fact, working memory and attention, in their presentation, share some features. In Joe's case, the focus is on attention, because his failure to remember the order is traced to his difficulty paying attention to key elements when he is stressed.

> *The best solutions?* A combination of environmental modifications and skill development.

• When a combination of sustained attention and working memory is involved, the first step is to modify the information-processing demand. There are three options: slow the information down; decrease the amount of information; repeat the information. This will aid both attention and working memory. If the attention problem stems from distractibility, as in the example here, repeating the information or decreasing the amount of information can help. In other situations, like trying to study, if possible eliminate the distraction or move to a place where it is not present and use an auditory or vibration prompt from a smart phone app to remind you to attend.

• Holding information in working memory requires storing it in the first place, which requires attention. The reason the "repeat" intervention will help Joe with attention is that having an intention in advance to repeat the order helps him focus specifically on this information to begin with. Repeating it covers both the attention and working memory issues since either he attends and gets it right or he gets it right by correction. Over time, his focus on this element is likely to improve.

> **Planning**—The ability to create a road map to reach a goal or to complete a task. It also involves being able to make decisions about what's important to focus on and what's not important.

JT: *Hey, you guys ready for Friday?*

MOM: *Always ready for the weekend, only 24 hours! Dad and I can't wait!*

JT: *Can't wait?*

MOM: *Can't wait; It's going to be so much fun!*

JT: *Glad you're psyched, didn't know you enjoyed performing.* (Laughs.)

MOM: *Performing? What are you talking about?*

JT: *Yeah, Friday night, some people are coming over, coworkers, boss might come. We were going to grill out. I texted Dad yesterday about it.*

MOM: *Did you hear back from him?*

JT: *Not yet. Why?*

MOM: *We're going to Sheryl's for the weekend. Her nephew is deploying; they're having a party. Your grandmother is coming to the house to take the dog. The house is getting mold work done on the walls from when the ice melt leaked in last winter. You told us you were going away with Sam.*

JT: *Oh, okay . . . That fell through; we didn't look for a hotel in time. So we'll be on our own cooking wise?*

MOM: *And housing wise. The mold removal involves fogging the house; it has to sit for 24 hours after, part of the reason we won't be there. I thought you said the trip with Sam was definite.*

JT: *It was. I didn't actually book it, though, and didn't know what it would cost or how far away the place was. It's like 4 hours one way. Where am I going to stay?*

MOM: *Not sure. You should probably figure it out soon, though. Love you!*

This scenario is a good example of two things: bad planning and how more than one executive skill can influence a real-life event. To echo the Captain in *Cool Hand Luke*, "What we've got here is a failure to communicate." Obviously JT and his mother aren't on the same page, but looking at each side of the discussion reveals one who is on top of the planning aspect and another who is not. The mother's texts indicate she has good planning skills; she knows what's happening, made provisions for the dog, and orchestrated a necessary and intrusive home repair to occur during a vacation. The assumptions JT has made aren't misplaced; there's no crime of ignorance in thinking on any given weekend his parents will be around the house. The problem is creating a situation in which he was dependent on that for multiple reasons that he didn't verify were feasible until it was too late. Some organization and time management could be playing into this, but the principal issue is planning, in this case poor planning. He didn't procrastinate or have a complete lack of direction, but he crafted a plan with several dependent factors, with a short time window, and executed it out of order.

> *The best solutions?* Environmental modification plus skill building. Once a tentative plan to reach a goal has been formed, before taking any steps to implement the plan, the plan originator needs to ask and answer the question "Does my plan involve any object, location, or person(s) over which I have no control?" If the answer is "yes," then permission must be sought and granted in advance to use the resources needed for the time period during which the plan will be carried out. If the resources are people, then their availability, absence, or permission must be confirmed. This solution requires the skill of initiation by the planner and in this case environmental supports required by the plan.

• First, if a tentative, different plan is on the table (e.g., JT's weekend trip), make a definite yes–no decision and inform any interested parties (including, in this case, the parents since they assumed this plan was in place).

• Second, before inviting people to a specific venue, make sure the venue is available (in this case, the house). Call Mom to check on the house availability, *then* invite coworkers. Booking a venue before you sell tickets seems fairly straightforward on the outside, but it takes practice to develop the foresight that prevents one from creating plans based on many assumptions.

> *The best overall fix is to set a rule for any plan that involves other people and/or specific locations:* Before proceeding with the plan, ask

about (1) the availability and willingness of other people to participate in the plan or (2) about the availability of and permission to use the venue.

• Since parents are often on the receiving end of a young adult's unspoken agenda, they are in a unique position to play the role of an environmental modifier.

> **Organization**—The ability to create and maintain systems to keep track of information or materials.

"Hey, Teg, did you get that e-mail out to State Management and Resources about income-based student loan payments?"

"Did I? Not yet. Was there an e-mail from them? Was it to my school or regular e-mail?"

"Not sure. I had you forward it to me a couple weeks ago. I can check my e-mail."

"Okay, yeah, 'cause my school e-mail, I tried to forward it to my personal account, but it got messed up and now some things go to the spam, some get pushed to the social bin—it's kind of a mess."

"Yeah, I can get it for you. Do you want the Netflix password too? For the documentary assignment?"

"Yeah, Dad, that sho—, wait, is it Netflix or Hulu or Amazon? Hold on, I bookmarked the page earlier." Tegan flipped through her phone. "Shoot, I guess I'm not signed in on my browser on my phone, so it's not coming up."

"So just grab your computer."

"I can't, my charger is missing and it's out of power. I think maybe I left it at work on Friday."

"Uhh, okay. Well, is there any way to recover those? You have to submit the loan payment form online by Sunday night to qualify; otherwise you're going to have to keep paying at the rate you were before. Which would sort of kill any chance of renting an apartment."

"Uhhhh, I think all my passwords are saved on my computer, so it means I'll have to reset the password for the state website and reset my e-mail password also."

"K, well, you should probably do that. Like I said, there's no time left to change it if you want to lower the payments."

The bright spot in Tegan's cascade of disorganization is that there is a way to salvage the device access and then the information that she needs. The downside comes in the few hours on the phone and help chats required to verify her ownership of the accounts. As is the case for many of us, Tegan's organizational issues involve both information (passwords, e-mail, websites) and objects (power cords). While sometimes things can be permanently lost, more often than not the downstream effect is search time, resulting in missed deadlines, late appointments, or inefficient problem solving. Device vulnerability aside (power outages, hackers), the growing reliance on smart phones and computers for information storage and access is a potential boon for people with weak organization.

> *The best solutions?* Environmental modifications. In this case, offloading information to a reliable source and location and use of location technology. Both are primarily environmental modifications, which usually carry the load in a skill weakness like organization.

• Password problems (misplaced, forgotten) are ubiquitous, universally so for people with organization problems. While passwords still dominate, there is growing use of fingerprints, retinal scans, facial recognition, and so on, as substitutes, and this potentially eliminates the problem of lost passwords. Easy availability of cloud storage and some of the accompanying organizational tools means that important information can potentially be accessed through any device, not simply the one you own. For example, using a password storage app to contain all passwords in a secure location (e.g., Last Pass, Dashlane, Stickey Password) can help. Another involves giving the information to a reliable source, in this case a parent.

• Sooner or later, people with organization problems should offload objects to a set location. Object misplacement has a couple of possible fixes. One is a form of offloading where a central location is chosen for storage of important objects (phone, keys, power cord). How do you remember to do that? A combination of repetition and reminders. After picking a location and container (e.g., a basket), take 5–10 minutes to repetitively place key items there, in the basket, and then move them to another location in the house, then pick them up and put them back in the basket. On the last practice run, leave the items in the basket until you need them.

• The high-tech option is using tagging tiles attached to important, often misplaced items. These Bluetooth-enabled tags can be located using a smart phone. If the phone is misplaced, it can be located using another phone or device that it is synced with.

> **Time Management**—The capacity to estimate how much time one has, how to allocate it, and how to stay within time limits and deadlines. It also involves a sense that time is important.

6:55 P.M.: *"Hi, Ry, it's me. I'm leaving now and should be there in a few minutes."*

"Siobhan, our reservation is for 7:00, and there's no way you'll be here in a couple of minutes. I'm not sure we'll be able to get in! Just hurry up, I'll meet you in the lobby."

"What took you so long, Shi? It's almost 7:30!"

"Traffic, then parking, I didn't think about it being Saturday."

"Can I help you, sir?"

"Hi, the name is Weaver, we have a reservation."

"I'm sorry Sir, we couldn't hold your reservation. Saturday is our busiest night."

"What should we do, Ry?"

"Listen, Shi, I think it's best if we call this off for tonight. We need to talk, but not tonight. And you've got to get this together if you want our relationship to work. I can't keep doing this."

The issue seems like it should have an easy fix, but Siobhan can't get a handle on it. She feels like she's always late, whether it's for a date, picking up her brother at school, or getting to appointments. And paying bills? Forget it. She's the queen of late notices.

Siobhan decides to focus on two areas. She really wants to build her relationship with her boyfriend, but it is obvious from the dinner fiasco that he is increasingly frustrated with her. And overdue payments of bills are now costing her almost monthly late payments.

> *The best solutions?* A combination of environmental modifications, skill building, and incentives. The environmental supports involve external timekeeping and alarm systems since one's "internal clocks" are not currently reliable. The skill development involves the commitment to consistently use these devices and, most important, the commitment to act at the time the device signals.

• The most common issues in weak time management are accurate time estimation and a lack of time urgency in the face of deadlines. Typically, for people with this weakness, time is underestimated based on best possible circumstances with no extenuating factors. In addition, it is usually accompanied by a "just one more thing before I go" urge, which when followed takes longer than expected and further degrades the optimistic time estimate. The solution is using a more generous time estimate and an agreement to forgo "just one more thing" until after you arrive at your destination. If you arrive early, you have time; if not, you would have been late.

• For both time estimation and time urgency, another powerful intervention, an environmental modification, is the person or institution on the receiving end of your tardiness holding you responsible. For example, your date cancels the date, you pay a significant late fee, lose service, and so on.

• Finally you can't rely on your internal sense of time as a prompt to leave. Audible alarms play a key role in your success.

• In her estimations of the travel time to get to dates, appointments, for example, Siobhan does not consider extenuating circumstances (traffic, time of day). For her, the simplest fix is to add 5 minutes for every 10-minute increment in her estimated travel time. For example, if she thinks a trip will take 30 minutes, she adds 15 minutes. Then, using the 45-minute travel estimate, at least 1 hour before she is to leave, she sets a series of alarms on her phone with the last being the "drop-dead" departure time that will give her the 45 minutes. If she'd like an added incentive, treating herself and her boyfriend to a weekend away, contingent on a certain number of on-time or early arrival for dates, is an option.

• To address on-time bill payment, she decides to try the TeuxDeux app on her phone, which lets her set up a day, time, and time frame with reminders to pay bills.

> **Goal-Directed Persistence**—The capacity to have a goal, follow through to the completion of the goal, and not be put off or distracted by competing interests.

"Dad, I think I need to pull $150 out of this month for expenses."
"Okay. For what?"
"For what? For bon bons, for doodads, for dongles and widgets. For what? If you need an invoice, leave a message on my extension at work."

"Haha, okay, fair enough. But in general, this is a problem for you, or could be. The point was to simulate paying rent, then dump the money into student loans or use it on a security deposit."

"No, I know, I know. But I am using this money for things that I need. I feel like part of my time living here is also about being able to spend the money that I need to, so when I move out I have what I need and am not scraping to buy stuff."

"And that's a good point. But what's the ultimate goal here? Sometimes I think you think that you're going to just transition into an apartment and have the exact same life you do here. But it isn't going to be that way. It isn't just the cost of the apartment, food, laundry, heat. It costs money, real money, and not always the same amount. So if the goal is a lifestyle, then maybe look for a roommate scenario. If the goal is your own place, then I think your argument that you can somehow prep for a time when you will have less money isn't as well thought out as you think. It's going to mean giving other things up."

"Dad, you know I value your opinion. But my goal is to be independent. Having a roommate isn't part of that for me, and actually making my own financial decisions is part of it. I'm planning by taking advantage of my situation now to prepare for later. I don't understand why that doesn't make sense to you."

"Because your goal isn't a goal; it's a bunch of goals that don't play well with one another. This kind of abstract, symbolic finish line is part of what puts you in these situations; the 'goal' is poorly defined, so you don't know how to reach it, so you don't really make any progress."

"Whatever. I'll give you $450 tomorrow, and if we can I'd like to drop the subject."

"Fine."

We frequently encounter money problems as a component of executive skills, in part because money raised for one purpose can easily be used for another. At the core of the goal-directed persistence problem, and the money problem, is the issue of deferral, saving versus spending, forgoing what I want today in favor of getting something better 3 days, 3 months, or 3 years from now. Making that future goal as "real" as possible allows it to compete with the immediately gratifying choice.

The best solutions? A combination of skill building and environmental modifications.

• These types of scenarios, involving the issue of immediate versus delayed gratification, arise regularly for young adults who struggle with GDP (goal-directed persistence). Effective exercise of this skill depends on the ability to ignore the present in favor of actions toward the long-term goal. An environmental modification such as aid from another person to help compensate for the weakness offers an advantage since it relies on that person's stronger GDP. That doesn't prevent the desire for immediate gratification from arising. That's why, noted below, clear expectations and rules about limits as well as about management of disagreements are key. In addition, since expenses are based on future projections, the young adult must develop a realistic expense plan, including establishing a "rainy day" reserve to adjust for unanticipated expenses. The restraint in this skill only develops with practice. Having short-term goals that are more easily achieved can help the young adult see the payoff in delay. Hence SMART goals that have short time horizons and offer small rewards are an important element in developing this skill.

• This involves establishing a high degree of specificity about the goal, matching it against current resources, deciding if the resources are sufficient, how they might need to be supplemented, and whether the effort needed is worth the payoff. There is a definite skill component in this process that involves planning as well as persistence. There is also a need for environmental support in the form of accurate, reliable information about the real "costs" of the goal. The availability of a person to consult with, such as a rental agent, helps to keep you from underestimating these real costs or overestimating your resources.

• If your goal is independent living in an apartment of your own, then job one is an accurate accounting of the real costs—security deposit, last month's rent, heat, utilities, food, and any "must have" creature comforts such as cable TV. (In the Appendix under "Locating and Costing Out an Apartment," we have detailed how to obtain these costs.)

• Match these costs against current income, savings, and expenses. This figure sets the savings plan as well as what current expenses need to be adjusted if the goal is to be reached. It also helps to determine if the goal is even attainable and, if it is, what sacrifices and compromises will need to be made.

• This clarifies what the young adult and the parent are prepared to do. Is a roommate acceptable? Is the parent willing to provide a rent subsidy to enable the single occupancy that the young adult thinks will be beneficial? Can the young adult and parent come to an agreement regarding what the monthly contribution will be and what options are there if the agreement is not met?

> **Flexibility**—The ability to revise plans in the face of obstacles, setbacks, new information, or mistakes. It relates to an adaptability to changing conditions.

"Dee, how goes the apartment hunt? Your dad and I aren't trying to get rid of you, but the space in this condo is pretty tight."

"I told you selling the house was a mistake! If we still had it, this wouldn't be an issue at all."

"With your dad and I retiring, Dee, you know we needed to pare down our expenses."

"Whatever! It wasn't my choice."

"C'mon, Dee, before we sold the house we talked about it, and you said you understood and even looked forward to having your own place."

"That's true, Mom, but I've been trying, and nothing has come up."

"Maybe you need to broaden your search area and criteria. Rents are more expensive here, and one-bedrooms are not the only option. What about other towns or even a roommate? I'll help however I can, but we really need you to move on this."

"Mom, I can't talk about this anymore now. I'll do what I can."

With some time to think about it, Dee realizes that her mom has a point.

For people like Dee, with flexibility weaknesses, the trigger issue is change. If she had her druthers, the family would still be in their house and everything would be fine for her, the operative words being "for her." With that option gone, she constructs a picture of the next best thing, a comfortable apartment that is affordable and close by. It's not home, but it's close. She fixates on that picture, unwilling to consider anything else. Without some insistence from her mother, she'd likely stay with them.

> **The best solutions?** Environmental modification plus skill building.

• A weakness in flexibility is challenging for a few reasons. For individuals with this weakness, change is experienced as a threat, and the greater the deviation from what is familiar, the greater the anxiety. In addition, there is a tendency to see the person or institution proposing the change as being at fault for causing the problem. Self-awareness of this weakness is particularly helpful since it opens the possibility of learning strategies to prepare for change and even deliberately exposing yourself to small changes. Practice with change in small doses increases flexibility.

• If you struggle with inflexibility, change can become easier for you if, whenever possible, you know about any change in schedule, plans, living arrangements, for example, well in advance of the change date. It is entirely reasonable to explain to family, friends, and colleagues that unexpected changes stress you out and that whenever a change is anticipated, it would help you if they could give you a heads-up in advance.

• Another aid is to introduce any major changes either you need to make or that other people need you to make in small steps.

• A third strategy is to include some choices in how the change takes place even in terms of time frames. Knowing what is coming, predictability, gives one a sense of control. Mental rehearsal of the change is especially helpful because each time you do it, the newness of the change is reduced.

• Last, having someone you're comfortable with accompany you through the change can make it easier.

> **Metacognition**—The ability to stand back and take a bird's-eye view of yourself in a situation. It is the ability to observe how you problem-solve. It also includes self-monitoring and self-evaluative skills (e.g., asking yourself "How am I doing?" or "How did I do?").

Chip sat down at the corner table of the cafe-style break room after clocking out for some leftover Chinese food. He dug in with one hand while pulling out his phone with the other, flicking through box scores and texts, waving the phone as Rob, the IT guy, pulled in a chair across from him.

"B's won."

"For real? I didn't see it. After the home run in the sixth I thought it was over for sure. Had to come in early today to check some stuff."

"Booker got you guys working 24/7 again? Damn, that sucks."

"Naw, it's not like that. Cory and I are building a new client app for sales, something we came up with on our own, couple hours a week in the morning. Probably take it to Booker in a few weeks. You know how I want to transfer over to Upton; I think this could put me over the top instead of waiting another 6 months."

"Oh, wow, that's cool, man. I wish Booker had something like that for me, something I could sink my teeth into here. I remember I talked to Jay a while ago about us talking to Booker about an idea we had to help improve sales at some of the accounts."

"Oh yeah? What happened with that?"

"Oh, nothing, really, just kind of fell off. You know, the company lost one of them before we got anything solid together, and then I was like 'What's the point?' You know?"

"Yeah, man." Rob looked around the room. "But there's still a point in it, though, you know? If it's a good idea, it's a good idea; there's a place and time for it somewhere. Why not run it by Booker now since there's still one account? Booker is all about better sales."

"Yeah, I guess you're right." Chip put the rest of his food in the refrigerator, said goodbye to Rob, and headed back to his desk, stopping midway to show Rob something about the box score and suggesting maybe talking to Booker.

Metacognition is about being able to step back, look at your performance in a situation, and use that information as a way to accomplish some goal. We all have moments in our lives we reflect on later as mistakes, or missed opportunities, or times when we made a course correction and really succeeded in achieving something significant. So, metacognition is a way to inform our future behavior. In this scenario, Chip is skilled in his field but treading water at a job he neither hates nor loves. He is presented with Rob as an example of someone who uses his skills and initiative to improve his circumstances. Chip tried this at one point, but when that specific idea didn't fit in that specific scenario, he gave up trying. Rob's actions should show Chip not only that the company responds to employee initiative but that it is possible to tailor the response to what satisfies your needs, in this case a location change rather than a promotion. This should have set off some bells in Chip's head, but it's not clear it did. This is a pattern of Chip's behavior that limits his mobility even though he's a talented individual with a lot to offer. He doesn't readily see his performance as lacking initiative (metacognition) and also doesn't see the different possibilities that his ideas might lead to. But Rob's final comment, feedback to Chip about taking action, may have set off some bells that didn't ring earlier.

The best solution? Environmental modification plus skill building.

• The key to metacognition is recognizing you have a problem. If this skill is a weakness, the most effective way to ensure problem recognition or good performance is to ask for performance feedback. One source of information that doesn't involve another person is a thorough review of your job description along with a blank copy of the company performance review form, assuming your company uses one. Typically, these reviews include the behaviors that the company expects from an employee. You can use this as a template to evaluate your performance. To get as accurate an assessment as possible, for each question try to think of specific examples of how you have met that expectation. The best source of this information is a supervisor or team leader. The approach goes something like this: "Karen, I've been working here a few months now. I'm really enjoying the work and being part of this company. I'm wondering if I could set up a time to meet with you for a kind of informal performance review. I want to be sure I'm doing the best work I'm capable of, and if there are areas to improve, I can work on those."

• For Chip, the information comes first from his colleague Rob. If he follows through on Rob's advice, there will be added information about Chip's idea/performance from his manager Booker.

• The skill component is learning to initiate or seek the feedback by asking, "How am I doing?" or "What can I do to improve my performance?" In his case, Chip initiated an idea but dropped it without any outside feedback. The conversation with Rob has at least opened the door for further initiation.

> **Stress Tolerance**—The ability to thrive in stressful situations and to cope with uncertainty, change, and performance demands.

"Hey, Mom."

"Wanda! This is unexpected! We just saw you on Friday! I don't mean I'm unhappy to see you, just a little surprised.'

"Yeah, I had some time, so I thought I pop in."

"Well, I'm glad, and your dad will be happy; he misses you. How're you doing? Is everything okay?"

"For sure, Mom, work is great and Karen is good, although I don't see her a lot; she stays with JT."

"What about Roxanne?"

"Yeah, she's around; we don't hang out much."

"Honey, are you a little homesick? In the last 2 months you've visited more than when you first moved."

"No, no, Mom, not at all! I really like having my own place, it's just that . . . "

"Just that . . . ?"

"That Roxanne is a drama queen! To hear her tell it, her life jumps from one emotional crisis to another. I've become her shoulder to cry on or confessor or therapist. I want to be a friend and support her, but there's no *end in sight. It's at the point that when I'm at my place, waiting for her to burst through the door sets my teeth on edge.*

"Well, what about your room as a safe haven?"

"Tried it. She either waits till I come out or knocks on the door."

"Wanda, you've always prided yourself on being there for friends, even going back to high school, helping them manage their crises. But you've got a lot on your plate right now, moving, new job, being on your own. Maybe you need some personal space for you."

"Yeah, but how do I get Roxanne to understand?"

Wanda has bumped into one of the major sources of stress, a form of "caregiver fatigue." While she is not, in the career sense, a caregiver, she has occupied this role informally for a good part of her life. Many people embrace and achieve great satisfaction from this role of helping others, as long as they have the time to do it. Stress enters the picture when they have their own needs to be met and/or there is no respite from the demand. Both are true for Wanda.

The best solutions? Environmental modifications and skill building.

• Creating boundaries that can be physical (such as one's room with the door closed) or communicative ("I don't want to discuss this topic"). The former is an environmental modification but still involves improving the skill since the barrier must be set and used consistently. The latter is more skill-based. In either case, deciding to create a boundary can be easier than maintaining it, especially for caregivers or friends when it involves a personal relationship. In some situations involving stress, environmental modifications such as avoiding the stressful event are effective management techniques. But it is not effective if the source of the stress is an ongoing presence in a place that the person cannot avoid. In addition, individuals with a weakness in stress management are susceptible to the ongoing stressors that accompany daily living, so it's important to learn stress-management strategies that can be used as a set of portable tools that can be applied across situations as they arise.

• To be successful Wanda will need to decide in advance what the boundaries will be. In this situation, she will need to have clear limits and expectations. This means eliminating herself as the "shoulder to cry on" or "therapist."

• As part of the conversation with Roxanne, Wanda, after she has set her own boundary, can offer to brainstorm resources that Roxanne might use. It will be best if Roxanne has a specific plan for who she will contact or what she will do.

• Since Roxanne is very likely to try to engage Wanda, Wanda needs to decide exactly what she will do and tell Roxanne. Her action needs to be specific and involve not attending to Roxanne. For example, she might go to her room, put on headphones, or go for a walk.

• The success of the plan depends entirely on Wanda sticking to it consistently.

• Wanda should anticipate that Roxanne will be upset and will direct her feelings toward Wanda to "blame" her. When this happens, Wanda needs to be firm in her resolve to maintain the boundaries she has set.

Taking Stock

Now is a good time to step back and briefly assess where you both are. If you've followed the steps of the process to this juncture, is there evidence of continued progress toward independence? Before you definitely answer this question, we offer a reminder or word of caution. "Progress toward" means just that, a work in progress, not a completed job. (If you're considering trying to use measures against baseline—money, chores, etc.—keep in mind that there's no absolute for this. The better assessment is whether there is continued movement.) If the young adult has followed the process of long-term goal setting followed by writing SMART goals to Step 8, one measure of progress is successfully reaching those SMART goals. If you feel that a SMART goal (or goals) has not been reached, review the SMART goal using the Step 6 evaluation form (page 175).

If the SMART goals criteria appear to have been met, but the goal has not been achieved, then the next phase is to look at the strategies for goal adjustment detailed in Step 7. But perhaps you want to answer the question that is more fundamental to the point of this book: Is the young adult making tangible, ongoing progress toward independence? The answer to that question can be found in a comparison of where the young adult started at the beginning of this process and where he is now using concrete markers of independence. The following questions provide a sample of the markers that signal independence.

Does the young adult now provide or has he or she achieved any of the following that were not present at the start of the process?

☐ Regular payments to you (e.g., from employment)? _____

☐ If yes, how much weekly? _____

☐ Pay own expenses? Rent _____ Spending money _____
Transportation _____ Clothing _____ Personal care items _____
Cell phone plan _____ Other _____

☐ Consistent help with household chores if living at home?
Laundry _____ Dishes _____ Cleaning _____ Shopping _____
Cooking _____ House repairs _____ Other _____

☐ Improvement in employment or career status? Working if not previously employed _____ Increase in wages _____
Work promotion _____ Career change or advancement _____

☐ Completion of an apprenticeship, training program, or degree necessary for job advancement or career entry? If yes, specify _____

☐ Are you and your young adult in agreement that progress has been made and is continuing? _____

☐ Are you and your young adult continuing to collaborate? _____
If not, has the young adult moved ahead and is he or she managing on his or her own? _____

If you've followed the steps in the process and, in spite of the efforts you and your young adult have made, you feel that progress toward independence has stalled and/or you are at an impasse, we have provided strategies to restart progress in Step 9.

STEP 9

··

Seek Extra Help If You're Still Stalled

How's it going? If you and your young adult had to answer that question, would you both say that progress is being made? That the designated goals in the plan are being met on time, or you've tweaked them to revise the plan so that forward motion has been restored? Remember our definition of independence. If skills and functioning that make the young adult more self-sufficient than before the Step 6 plan was in place are developing, the plan is working. Keep going!

What if you two disagree? Have you yielded to the temptation to push for faster progress, either ignoring problems with the original timeline or goal definition or pushing to exceed what's written in the plan? Is the young adult claiming success without concrete, measurable evidence that it's being achieved? If one of you is satisfied with what's being accomplished and one isn't, revisit Steps 5 and 6 to remind yourselves of the goals and the agreed-on plan for reaching them. If, as a result, you decide progress is lagging, first revisit what you've learned in this book:

- Check the Executive Skills Questionnaires you two filled out in Step 1 and Step 4. Have you underestimated the impediments caused by an executive skills weakness in the young adult? Have you two relied on parental assistance where the parent is actually weak in the same executive skills as the young adult? Review the creative ideas for dealing with specific skill weaknesses in Step 8.

- Are you sure you, the parent, are providing support that really supports rather than coerces? Review Step 2 if you need a reminder of what

222

coercion looks like. Are you subtly sabotaging the young adult's efforts because you don't really believe in the goal or the plan? Remember our cautions about letting the young adult make the decisions, including the goal and action step plans, and review our advice in Step 5. Use collaborative communication à la the tips in Step 4 to come to agreement.

- Has the young adult tried to work toward a goal that is beginning to look like a stretch, but both of you are trying to spare the young adult feeling like he's failing (yet again)? If you're the young adult, consider redoing the GTKMQ in Step 3. Maybe you can identify an alternative or less ambitious course that still fits with your interests and aptitudes.

- Is the young adult being thwarted by the same types of pitfalls on every action step, and she's getting worn out by trying to do damage control and makeup work? Go back to the ideas in the three tables in Step 7 and see if you can find some unexplored tools to use.

> *If progress is lacking, review your journey through the preceding steps to see if there's anything you've missed or want to go over again.*

What If the Young Adult Is Stuck at Square One?

The preceding list is predicated on the idea that young adults and parents have actually gotten through Steps 1–8—not just reading the material but doing the work to identify capacities and interests, determine readiness and motivation, gather support, set a goal, make a plan, and start taking action. But what if you've read through all those steps and the young adult hasn't even figured out what he wants to and can do?

Interest and Motivation: Linchpins for Change

While each of the young adults we've described so far has a different starting point, the catalyst for movement for each is an interest in a goal that serves as the vehicle of motivation. In a couple of the cases, for example, Trafina and Casey, the interests were already known but they needed to identify a path that coincided with their preferences and skills. And both benefited from the support of parents in allowing them to continue in their current living situation while they made tentative but tangible movement toward a goal. In Trafina's case, she needed executive skills support. In Casey's situation, he accommodated an executive skills weakness by choosing a learning environment that compensated for his executive skills weaknesses, and his parents were willing to support this. For Jonas, the impetus to move came in part from his mother, and he pursued what was initially a vague interest but something they both could tolerate since it fit with his other interests. In addition, he chose a set of circumstances that accommodated his executive skills weaknesses and he profited from his mother's executive skills support when he ran into some initial obstacles. For Cheyenne, the impetus to move came more from social awareness of her peers moving forward. She benefited from working collaboratively with her dad in using his executive skills to explore an interest area that became clearer once she was able to identify her personal preferences and skills.

Of the four young adults, it would be fair to say that only Trafina had an existing passion, her interest in art. For the others, perhaps their interests will become passions over time, but for now the opportunity to develop a skill in an area of interest that also holds out the possibility of career advancement is sufficiently motivating to maintain a degree of momentum. We emphasize the importance of this because for many young adults that we meet the admonishment of commencement speakers at high school and college graduations that emerging young adults "follow their passion" can trigger unspoken anxiety.

What happens when you don't have a passion? Do you follow your peers into some type of postsecondary education in the hopes that you'll discover some dormant or latent passion? Or if you or your parents don't have the resources to afford this opportunity, do you drift from situation to situation and job to job assuming that this will reveal your passion? As parents we should not be surprised at this uncertainty considering that, even for the typical young adult, executive skills don't fully develop until about age 25. Moreover, self-awareness in the form of metacognition, goal planning, and goal-directed persistence are the last of these skills to develop. For emerging young adults with a history of weaknesses in metacognition, flexibility in behavior and thinking, planning, task initiation, and sustained attention, the problem is that much more exaggerated. As a result, they are more at risk for what appears to parents as aimless drifting and a sense of uncertainty, which is, in fact, what it is. The result is a period of prolonged young adulthood that parents, for what seem or what are legitimate reasons, may feel obligated to support.

How long should this go on? If the process of discovering an interest can happen in a reasonable, timely fashion, it's well worth the investment of effort and time on the part of the young adult, parents, or anyone else who can provide outside guidance and information. The potential payoff in discovering an interest is its impact as a catalyst for motivation and self-determination by the young adult, and potential attainment of a goal that will result in increased independence. The operative word here is "timely." Because of the variability in young adults' situations, we can't define a hard-and-fast time frame or limit for this process. However, we would note that without intending it, young adults and parents can slip into a pattern of support where weeks easily stretch into months and perhaps years. Shayleigh's mother and stepfather saw the potential for this to happen. Dylan's parents did too, even though their son had agreed to a particular SMART goal.

> *Every situation is different, but for young adults who are trying to discover an interest, it's probably wise to review and change the game plan as necessary after about 3 months.*

In cases like these, a 3-month review seems quite reasonable. If your young adult has made no progress toward a plan or a job and is not contributing in a meaningful way to the household, it is time that you mutually agree to SMART goals that target increased self-sufficiency with short time horizons. If the process sputters, the discussion that follows may provide some direction. First, though, let's take a look at how Dylan's parents and Colin's (my wife and I) approached this kind of obstacle.

Dylan

Dylan's situation epitomizes what can happen when a young adult is stuck but well enough supported to be comfortable in his stuckness. Dylan persisted neither with school nor with work and has settled into a fairly passive but comfortable lifestyle with support at home.

Where he started: We met Dylan when he was living at home and neither working nor attending school, completely dependent on his parents for support. He evidenced no self-initiated desire to move out of this situation. His eventual impetus to start was a push from his parents that he needed to work or go to school.

Where he wanted to get to and why he was stuck: Dylan was content to continue with the status quo, and he had no particular interest other than video games, to which he had unfettered access. He identified weaknesses in task initiation and goal-directed persistence as well as a situational weakness with sustained attention if he wasn't interested in the task. Under pressure from his parents, Dylan identified cybersecurity as something he might be interested in and agreed to pursue information about course work in this area.

Was the goal a good fit? To the extent that cybersecurity related to computers, it was potentially a good fit. The one other potential advantage of school was that other than setting aside a time for an online class, Dylan's current life-style did not need to change. However, Dylan chose this option under pressure from his parents, and he had previously not expressed any particular interest in this area. Thus, both his questionable motivation and executive skills weaknesses were potentially significant impediments to good fit.

What support did he need to reach his goal? Dylan needed financial support to take the course, and his parents agreed to provide the support if Dylan did the initial leg work to determine what steps he would need to take for course work and a cybersecurity certificate.

Did he reach his goal? Together Dylan and his parents set up a SMART goal involving a limited time period for Dylan to independently gather information about the course of study. Dylan failed to meet this initial SMART goal, and his parents took the school option off the table.

What's next? Dylan needs to demonstrate some basic life skills as a way to compensate for and justify the unconditioned support that his parents are currently providing. Since the impetus is coming from his parents, they identify two areas. One is the consistent performance of a set of chores at least 3 days a week that will assist with the family routines. The second area is initiation of a job search, including identification and application for entry-level work. His parents realize that Dylan will need some incentive to complete this, and since playing online games is the most motivating activity that Dylan has, they make access to the Internet on the computer contingent on two factors: completion of the chores and concrete demonstration of the results of his job search with applications submitted. Dylan suspects that this is a limit that his parents will not follow through on, but after 4 days of no access to the Internet Dylan agrees to begin with his chores and the job search. He is initially inconsistent in his completion of chores, but Internet access is contingent on day-to-day chore completion, and once he realizes this, he becomes consistent. As an added incentive to locate and maintain employment, his parents tell Dylan they will give him the upcoming upgrade so he can have the smart phone he wants. However, they make access to service contingent on his maintaining satisfactory employment.

Colin

Colin's executive skills weaknesses include task initiation, sustained attention, and time management. At one point, I thought his goal-directed persistence was weak also but realized this was only the case if he was uninterested in the tasks or goal. College, in selected areas, fell into that category. Subsequent to his freshman year struggles and suspension, he tried school again with a continuing pattern of hits and misses, doing well in some subjects and failing others. Realizing that a degree was a distant long shot, he left school and went to work landscaping in Nantucket.

Where he started this phase: After nearly 2 years in Nantucket, Colin returned home. While he had no definite interests or goal in mind, he discovered that Nantucket was not for him. The island had its benefits in terms of its physical attractions and a well-paying, stable job where he could have advanced. But neither the locale nor the type of work held the draw that it initially had for him. My wife and I were happy to see him home since we had seen little of him over the past 2 years, and we had an in-law apartment downstairs where he and his sister had intermittently lived. He returned with sufficient savings to support himself for a while.

Where he wanted to get to and why he was stuck: His intent was to find work that was more intellectually stimulating and to relocate with a friend in Boston. He had a vague idea about getting an entry-level job in the publishing industry, but no definite strategy. Neither option materialized. He didn't find a job, and his friend was ambivalent about giving up the stability of living at home, so Colin remained at home too. In the interim he did some landscaping and construction work for us, and he picked up some intermittent work doing hazardous waste removal and abatement with his friend's father's company. From early April on he settled into this situation through the summer with no job and no real end in sight.

Was his goal a good fit? Colin had no burning interest or passion for any particular type of work, but since he liked writing, an entry-level position with a publisher was as good an option as any. But since he had no published work at that point and no degree, he had no real foot in the door.

What support did he have to reach his goal? Since writing was an interest for him and I was lead author on *Smart but Scattered Teens,* I asked if he would help with the book by writing the vignettes for the executive skills sections, a central component in the book. He agreed, and in exchange his compensation was our support for his living expenses and some spending money. He also decided that for a career with an intellectual bent he needed a degree and enrolled in an online bachelor's degree program, which we helped him fund since he had some money left over from leaving his job in Nantucket.

Did he reach his goals? For school he did not. He passed one course and withdrew from a second course and again set school aside. Regarding his interest in writing, procrastination aside, he wrote all of the vignettes and the parent questions/answer sections for eleven chapters of the teen book, covering all of the executive skills. This material constituted the essence of each chapter, and he received strong positive feedback from our editors. The book was completed the following March, and based on his significant contributions Colin became a coauthor on the book. He and his friend resurrected their plan to move to Boston with the promise of assistance for his rent from my wife and me. His continued search for publishing work yielded no results. While the teen book wasn't his goal and hadn't even been on his horizon, it yielded psychological and eventual financial benefits, and he was happy with his accomplishment.

What came next? Colin liked living in Boston, in part related to a new relationship with a woman there. But by the end of June he had still not found any work, and my wife and I were concerned that he had settled into a comfortable lifestyle with our support with no end in sight from our perspective. We realized that by providing support without any conditions or expectations we had created a situation where he was stalled but sufficiently content with his lifestyle that there was no sense of urgency about changing it. At that point we also knew that we needed to set some expectations. Not for the first time, however, we experienced that setting limits for a child that you love is difficult. It is especially difficult if you've been supportive for an extended period of time and sense that it will provoke some unhappiness in your child. But we bit the bullet and told him he needed to find a job in 3 weeks and that, one way or another, we were substantially reducing his rent support. For us, it was not a pleasant confrontation, and Colin was not happy with us, but he said that he understood and the conversation ended. As he seems to have a knack for accomplishing things when limits are set, he moved on, and within 2 weeks he had a job unloading fish at a fisherman's co-op. Based on his work ethic and his quiet ability to relate positively to people, in 6 weeks he moved from this job on land to working as a deckhand on a trawler at sea. For a month, to stabilize his finances, he worked both jobs and ridiculous hours. He fished for 13 months, which is where you met him in the Prologue, working on this book.

I offer this example to illustrate that even for someone who might know better, you can find yourself in a situation where as a parent, with good intentions, you've played a role in your adult child being stuck.

Providing the Impetus for Change

As illustrated by Dylan and Colin, the impetus must originate with you if you expect the situation to change. The struggle, as we've mentioned many times, is that the impetus usually involves a change in the young adult's living circumstances, either decreasing the support or increasing the expectations in exchange for that support, or both. The change is not likely to be seen, at least initially, as a favorable one by the young adult. He may react with annoyance or anger or, if you overshoot the demand, anxiety about the loss of support, the safety net.

When you're the agent of some unhappiness for your child, you usually don't feel positive about it. (Unless, of course, you believe, "I know this hurts but in time you'll thank me for it." This may well be true, but in the moment it is little consolation.) For some parents, not wanting to make the adult child unhappy is enough to maintain the status quo. For others, the situation goes on until they reach a breaking point and opt for a "tough love" stance.

We favor a middle ground that leads to gradually increasing expectations and decreasing support (an approach we didn't quite manage with Colin). We also recommend a communication approach that frames the change as a reflection of reality. For example:

> "Dee, you've said that you want to make your own decisions about a direction to head in rather than us telling you what to do. We want that for you also. At the same time, we're also getting older, and Dad and I want to have the money to do things we planned when you and your brother grew up. He's pretty settled and we'd like to see you be able to move toward some goal and independence for yourself. We know you're not sure what direction you want to go in and you want to make that your choice, which we've supported. At the same time, it's been some time, and while you're deciding, we need you to start contributing financially and also helping us around the house. We didn't want to hit you with this all at once, but we thought it was better if you knew what we've been thinking about. We don't need you to do anything right now, so how about if you think it over and we can talk more specifically in a couple of days."

The approach is meant to avoid confrontation or threats and leave the young adult in charge of her own life, while at the same time presenting the realities of your own. Giving her a few days to think it over lets her know what's coming and gives her a chance to consider her options.

With these considerations in mind, let's review the central issues for you and your young adult if you find yourself in the situation where the young adult has no interest that acts as the catalyst for motivation and you are both caught in a state of suspended animation.

- The time period for the young adult's discovery of an interest needs to be limited, preferably with a defined endpoint.

- All things considered, a short time horizon is preferable. We suggested 3 months of no discernible progress or movement. (Dick here: My wife and I didn't follow this advice. Colin seemed happy and we didn't want to rain on his parade. Our mistake.)

- The critical goal is increased self-sufficiency and a move toward independence, preferably in two areas, life skills (shopping, money management, appointments, personal care, etc.) and employment. Regarding the latter, in the absence of an interest, you both accept the reality that *a* job is the important criterion, regardless of status. An interesting job offers more possibilities, but as with a vocational interest, the wait and/or search cannot go on indefinitely.

- Procrastination on the part of parent(s) contributes to and encourages procrastination in the young adult.

- Finally, if the expectations that you present to your young adult seem fair, stick to them and to the timelines you've set. If you're ambivalent, the young adult will be ambivalent.

Coaching

Sometimes young adults and parents are unable to establish goals that the young adult finds motivating and the parents can support. Parents may not have the resources or skills or young adults may not be comfortable with their parents' help. Or perhaps the young adult identifies a goal she wants to attain and the parent supports this goal but the young adult remains stuck. What's the option in this case? One option is outside help in the form of a coach.

What Is a Coach?

Traditionally, we think of a coach as a person who works with an athlete to help the athlete develop a set of skills and then apply those skills in a particular task or situation to achieve a goal. Along the way, the coach monitors the athlete's skill acquisition, provides corrective feedback when needed, and offers encouragement. Over the past 20 years we have developed and refined a coaching model to address goal setting and goal achievement for individuals with executive skills weaknesses.

Through our work, the model we've developed and similar models developed by others have been adapted for use with college students and with young adults and even older adults who are having difficulty with goal setting and attainment. In these models, the young adult and coach typically work together, with the coach taking on the following roles:

- The coach collaborates with the young adult to directly address and resolve problems that interfere with goal setting and goal attainment.

- The coach acts as a resource for the young adult when the parent is not able to provide the assistance.

- The coach serves as a "surrogate frontal lobe" to temporarily lend her or his executive skills to support the young adult's weak areas. This support is gradually reduced over time as the young adult becomes more practiced and proficient in using executive skills to attain goals.

We see two major components in the coaching process:

- The first involves the young adult and coach working collaboratively to build a relationship of trust and then helping the young adult establish a long-term goal. A long-term goal begins to shift the young adult's focus away from the immediate satisfaction and distraction of day-to-day activities and toward some future desired goal. When the young adult establishes a long-term goal and understands how his day-to-day behavior can affect that goal, he gets one step closer to regulating his behavior to serve the long-term goal (e.g., turning off the video game to complete a work or school assignment).

- The second is regular, recurring coaching sessions to help the young adult experience the connection between day-to-day behaviors and the attainment of his longer-term goal. Following this, the young adult, with guidance from the coach, learns and practices techniques (implementation intentions, mental contrasting, and simulation; see Step 7) that will build the executive skills behaviors necessary to accomplish short-term tasks that lead to a long-term goal.

When Is a Young Adult a Candidate for Coaching?

Coaching can be a fit for any young adult who wants to achieve a goal, recognizes there are impediments in the way, and is open to working with someone to bypass or resolve those impediments. Coaching is a process of collaboration and trust. Young adults may be understandably reluctant or skeptical about the process, but many of these doubts can be overcome by knowing what to expect. Following the description of the coaching process are some more ideas for creating openness to coaching.

The coaching services we are familiar with each have their own procedures, but they all include similar steps.

The Coaching Process

Coaching is designed to help young adults collaborate with a coach to set and achieve their own goals. The model has two phases:

- In phase one, the young adult and coach work together to develop a goal of the young adult's choosing and to work on specific plans to meet those goals.

- In phase two, the young adult and the coach meet on a regular basis to set short-term SMART goals, break down tasks to be accomplished, and develop strategies to anticipate and overcome any obstacles that might arise.

PHASE ONE

In the first session or two, the young adult and the coach meet and the coach describes, in general, what the coaching process involves. Sometimes this can be done on the phone or via social media. There are also a number of programs that offer online, distance coaching. This first phase offers an opportunity for the young adult to ask any questions or raise concerns to ensure that he is comfortable with the process. After this, the young adult and the coach discuss the young adult's background, including interests, special skills, past work experiences, and activities that the young adult enjoys participating in. This discussion would review the information that is contained in the GTKYQ. If the young adult has completed this questionnaire, he can take it to the first meeting with the coach. If the young adult has completed the Executive Skills Questionnaire, he can also bring it to the first meeting to discuss his pattern of strengths and weaknesses. Following that, the young adult and coach discuss what interest the young adult has in pursuing training, additional schooling, or a particular career. If the young adult has identified a strong interest or a tentative goal, he and the coach can begin mapping out a game plan for the steps needed to accomplish this goal. If the young adult has not identified any particular interest areas or possible long-term goal, he and the coach can look over his interests and subject areas in school and/or past work that he liked or disliked. Based on this information, they can brainstorm together possible interest areas and work together, using the coach's resources, to identify possible interests and the prerequisites needed to pursue them. The final component in this first phase is a discussion of the goodness of fit between the young adult's expressed interest or goals or how well these mesh with his current abilities, as well as the skills that he will need to acquire the prerequisites if he hasn't yet fulfilled those. The session ends with a discussion of any additional information that the young adult would like to acquire, as well as what the coach recommends that he bring to the next session, and they agree on a meeting time.

> Coaching can help the young adult arrive at a goal and then stay on track toward achieving it through regular meetings with the coach.

PHASE TWO

In regular coaching sessions, once a tentative goal has been established and the young adult and coach have collaborated on the steps to be accomplished to reach that goal, the remaining sessions are devoted to working on accomplishing these steps. These sessions constitute the heart of the coaching process, with each session focusing on establishing short-term SMART goals. The discussion includes the specific tasks that need to be accomplished, specific time frames for completing the tasks, and the criteria by which successful completion will be defined. The young adult and the coach mentally rehearse completion of each task in the process and identify any potential obstacles that may be encountered and the strategies that can be used to overcome these obstacles. As part of this process, the young adult and the coach discuss tools and supports that the young adult might find helpful in accomplishing the tasks. These might include smart phones, alarms, alerts, apps and text messages, e-mails, and phone contacts exchanged by the young adult and the coach to prompt and check progress. These are specified in a written plan that the young adult and coach have copies of. The young adult and coach will also specify the young adult's preferred method of contact and check-ins. In addition to specifying times when these will take place, the young adult and coach agree on the next face-to-face session, and the session ends. At the following session the young adult and coach will review the tasks that have been accomplished and trouble-shoot reasons that have prevented the young adult from completing her tasks, if there are any, and they will plan next steps. This process continues through the sessions. Coaching sessions are decreased in frequency or end when the young adult and coach are satisfied that the young adult has demonstrated that she can accomplish SMART goals independently.

NEED MORE INFORMATION?

See the Resources at the back of the book, where you'll find a list of web links with annotations of agencies for different areas of the country. Based on our professional experience, these services are well qualified to provide executive-skills-informed coaching.

Building Openness to Coaching

As we noted, trust and collaboration are essential in a coaching relationship. Therefore, coercion has no place in building a young adult's motivation to try it. No benefit is gained if parents try, in some fashion, to force their young adult to participate. However, we know that a key motivating factor for the young adult is a desire to move on. Hesitation is often caused by fear of failure. If there is tension or increasing conflict between parent and young adult and/or the young adult wants to be free of parent intrusiveness, this dissonance can also be an incentive. In opening the discussion about coaching, the parent can acknowledge wanting to help, not wanting more conflict, and being at a loss for how to proceed. Parents can also consider offering an incentive for giving the process a try. If the incentive is modest (we're not talking new cars here) and is tied to only a trial visit, the young adult is in a "take it or leave it" position. In our work, we do not view incentives as coercive. Beyond this, parents can point their young adult in the direction of coaching resources and leave the decision to her. If the young adult decides to engage in coaching, parents are not part of the process unless invited in by the coach or the young adult.

Finding a Coach

While coaching executive skills has been available for some years with high school and more recently with college students, it is a new and emerging inter-vention for young and older adults. How do you locate a coach? Other than the websites we have offered, we offer a note of caution about selecting a coach.

Life coaching has become the chosen profession for an increasing number of individuals. And a growing number of individuals and organizations offer training and certification credentials for coaching. As a result, the quality of the training and the credentials vary widely, as do the entry-level credentials of the coach. Executive-skills-informed coaching constitutes only a very small subset of this large coaching world, with fewer qualified coaches. However, given the growing knowledge of, interest in, and "marketability" of executive skills, some coaches may claim expertise in the area regardless of qualifications. One helpful resource is the "Tips for Finding an Executive Function Coach," published on the website of the Clay Center of Massachusetts General Hospital. This information can be found at the following web link: *www.mghclaycenter.org/ parenting-concerns/grade-school/executive-function-coaching.*

Tech "Coaches"

If you and your young adult are at an impasse and he does not want to participate in coaching or you are unable to find a coach, is there another option? In fact, technology in the form of smart phone apps and computer-based tools can be a viable and valuable source of help. As a population, we all have become increasingly reliant on technology to prompt and coach our behavior. Our cars tell us when we are out of our lane, too close to another car, and need to brake. In some cases, if we don't act, the car acts for us. And we depend increasingly on our smart phones or computers as devices where we can offload information and functions. They serve as what are described in the world of cognitive rehabilitation as "cognitive orthotic devices." As such, they can serve as highly effective compensatory tools for weaker executive skills. For young adults who are quite familiar with the value of technology since they have grown up with it, coaching and goal-setting apps are one more, nonjudgmental tool that are in many ways more reliable than a coach or parents since they can be consistent and ever-present. Coaching and goal-setting apps are readily available, and it's easy to use a search engine to identify those that are most suited to a particular young adult's needs—many are even rated for effectiveness.

Young adults who are interested in self-management should explore this option before considering more traditional coaching. Colin uses these resources on a daily basis as his "pocket coach." He recommends that young adults who are reluctant to work with a more traditional coach try these as a stand-alone resource or as an introduction to the benefits of in-person coaching. You'll find sources of more information about coaching programs in the Resources.

Young Adults and Psychological Issues

Stress is a common and expected feature of the transition to young adulthood. For the first time, young adults are facing the fact that sooner rather than later they will be on their own. While this can be appealing and exciting, it can also provoke anxiety. For the young adults we have discussed in this book, the stress in this transition is exacerbated. They are stuck, likely aware that they're stuck, and see no obvious way out. They have already experienced some failures in terms of attaining goals and often see them as personal failings that are accompanied by a sense of inferiority. The longer the situation goes on, particularly in the context of watching peers and friends move ahead, the more discouragement and anxiety are likely to increase. While these feelings are a natural part of the uncertainty that young adults face, how do parents and young adults know when these feelings reach a point that outside support may be needed? The behavioral markers for more significant anxiety and depression include the following:

- Reduced energy, especially if there is a corresponding increase in reduced activity. This could be manifested in difficulty getting out of bed, increased isolation, and a reduction in usual activities.

- Loss of interest in activities. Young adults may continue to participate in activities such as going out with friends, but express no enjoyment from these activities.

- Increased irritability and/or anger that represents a change in the usual disposition of the young adult.

- Verbal and nonverbal signs of hopelessness or sadness reflected in statements, crying, or facial expressions.

- Changes in eating and sleeping habits, either significant increases or decreases, and different from the young adult's typical baseline.

- Increases in risk-taking behavior, including substance abuse, sexual activity, and gambling, among others.

Regarding this last point, parents may well see or be aware of substance use, sexual activity, and gambling in their young adult. As we noted earlier, once young adults reach legal age, they are free to consume alcohol, use marijuana in states where it is legal, and engage in sexual activity with partners of their choosing. While parents may find these behaviors distressing or unacceptable to their values, for many young adults they are typical and not a cause for alarm. When should parents be concerned? When they see, on a daily basis, one or more of the preceding signs of anxiety or depression and/or excessive engagement in one of these behaviors. These include regular drug and alcohol intoxication, evidence of driving while impaired, marked weight loss or weight gain, sexual promiscuity, and excessive debt due to gambling or spending binges. For parents who have concerns about the behaviors of their young adults, we recommend the following:

• Seek advice from a licensed mental health professional, preferably from one who has experience with young adults, to determine if your concerns are warranted. Keep in mind that this is a discussion about your concerns and what you might do to change or improve the situation. Unless you have explicit, written permission from your young adult, you are not at liberty to reveal her personal or identifying information, and what you hear from the professional is advice about your feelings and behaviors, not indirect treatment for your young adult to pass on to her.

• If your concerns are warranted, the next step is to have a conversation with your young adult. It is not your role to offer an opinion about what you think her problem is or why it is occurring or your guess at a diagnosis or what she should do to resolve it.

• The most important action you can take when concerned about your young adult's behavior or emotional well-being is to express your concern about the young adult and your willingness to help in whatever way the young adult chooses. It is important that you approach the young adult with compassion and empathy and especially with respect for the fact that it is the young adult alone who makes the decision about what action to take.

• If the young adult indicates that you are part or the cause of the problem, offer to see a counselor alone or jointly with her, and when you do, share the outcome with her to the extent you are comfortable.

Often young adults, unless they have had past experience with a counselor, are not sure how to access help or what might be involved in the process. Providing them with information about counseling and resources in the community or where they might access such information gives them the option to think about it without committing to it. Let them know that seeing a counselor is an opportunity to talk with a trained person about one's thoughts and feelings and can help to relieve anxiety and stress.

If your young adult expresses no interest in taking some action or refuses to even discuss the subject, you need to accept this decision. This can be particularly difficult when you're worried about your child and concerned about his welfare. However, badgering or attempting to coerce him will make the situation worse and lower the chance that he'll seek any help. There is ample evidence that compassion, expressions of caring, and ongoing support from parents can be a significant protective factor for young adults. In the Miscellaneous Resources section in the Appendix at the end of the book, under Psychological Issues, we have provided a link to websites that provide guidelines for parents and for young adults with suggestions for support and ways to access resources.

STEP 10

··

Learn from Your Success

One of the greatest difficulties for young adults with executive skills weaknesses is learning from experience. That's because this type of learning is bestowed through the skill of metacognition, and it's one of the last to develop—often not until the mid-to-late 20s. Unfortunately, without adequate metacognition, young adults who have been stalled often stay that way, because they keep making the same mistakes. Even when they've begun to move forward, they're vulnerable to falling back into old patterns of behavior driven by other executive skills weaknesses, from the impulse spending that kept them ineligible to sign a lease, to the disorganization that led to lost keys and repeated lateness to work, to the lack of flexibility that fuels creative problem solving—a key to successful adult functioning. Without access to the bird's-eye view of metacognition, young adults don't reflect on their own experiences and often don't notice how others are reacting to them either, whether it's the boss's growing exasperation with their tardiness or the girlfriend's tiring of daily blow-ups.

Obviously suffering the consequences of the same mistakes over and over is demoralizing and slows progress toward goals. Just as great a hindrance, however, is failure to learn from successes. We all navigate life's land mines over time by learning what works for us as well as what doesn't. Recognizing our errors keeps us from slipping backward. But identifying the skills, behaviors, and strategies behind our successes helps us make strides forward.

In this final step on the journey toward independence, we want to highlight reflection, for both young adults and parents. We hope you've both learned approaches and strategies that have served progress well. Now we'll use the experiences of the young adults profiled in this book to illustrate how successful ways of working toward goals can be brought to the surface, labeled, and then used creatively to keep the positive momentum going.

Dylan

Dylan's stated goal of getting into cybersecurity met none of the criteria for good fit. Having been plucked out of the air when he was under pressure by his parents to come up with something to aim for, it matched neither his aptitudes nor really his interests, and the educational requirement ran afoul of his weaknesses in task initiation and goal-directed persistence. As we described in Step 9, he failed to research certification, and so his parents withdrew their offer of financial support for this educational pursuit. Dylan's parents wisely saw that Dylan needed an incentive to move forward, and so they tied access to his online gaming to modest goals of doing chores regularly and searching for a job. It took time, but doing chores became habitual once Dylan realized that his access to the pastime that gave him pleasure depended on persistent chore completion. His motivation to find a job was enhanced as well by his parents' buying him the new phone that optimized his gaming but making paying for monthly cell service contingent on Dylan's finding a job within 60 days and keeping it.

Dylan did find an entry-level job working at a call center for a bank, doing online searches, and providing customer information on account updates. But not simply because he wanted his parents to keep paying for his cell service so he could play his games anywhere. That required goal-directed persistence that was in short supply for him. His problems with task initiation also made it very challenging for him to even start his job search when he was doing it in the very same environment in which he had spent whole days (day after day) doing nothing but playing his games. He tried spending time at the local coffee shop but found there was no disincentive to shifting away from the job site to his game sites. Dylan's mother suggested that he do his job search at home and offered to come in and check on his progress every 10 minutes to reinforce goal-directed persistence. This solution felt like nagging to Dylan, who countered with the idea that he would do his job search in the same room as one of his parents while they were reading or working on their own computers (not watching TV or doing something else distracting). He thought just having a parent there would remind him to stick to the task, and he was right. Unfortunately, his attention still wandered. So he would find an interesting job lead and then drift off to some other thread and lose the job link. This meant that, even when he had spent an hour on job sites and come up with some promising leads, he wouldn't have any evidence of his efforts to show to his parents. His father nudged Dylan to take the initiative here and asked him if his new phone had any apps that he could use to issue reminders or give him a quick way to record the positive results he was producing. He found an app that would ask him every 10 minutes if he had recorded good leads and another one that would store them for later use in applying.

During his first few weeks at his new job, Dylan complained that it was boring and depended largely on his parents to wake him up in time for work and make sure he got out the door. His parents considered this assistance worth the payoff of seeing Dylan stick out the job, but after a month they decided it was time to withdraw such help. To transfer the responsibility of getting to work on time to their son, they offered to set up a shared account where they would match what Dylan put in the account to purchase a new, faster computer with an advanced graphics package.

Over the next 6 months Dylan realized that he liked the problem-solving aspect of his job involving customer questions and account management. His supervisor told him about the positive feedback the bank received in customer surveys about his work. He indicated that if Dylan continued his efforts he would be in line for a promotion.

Successful Strategies

• *Use incentives that tap into preferences.* When Dylan's parents tied his pleasures (gaming) to his achieving modest but concrete SMART goals, he started to recognize that his love of gaming was a powerful force in overcoming his executive skills weaknesses. He decided to set up his own schedule of gaming rewards (playing time, buying new games) for future goals. For example, when his boss asked him to write up his own performance review, he sat on it until he cut his usual gaming time by 30% nightly to get it done in increments over a week, with the reward of a new app when his review was completed and e-mailed to his boss.

• *Use tech tools to their maximum potential.* Dylan didn't have any coding or programming skills that were directly transferable to the job market, but his ability to dig up the best games was transferable to finding the best executive-skill-assisting apps available on his brand-new phone. In addition, the problem-solving skills he acquired in gaming were transferable to problem solving for customer questions about account management and bank services that they could use to their benefit.

Colin

When I returned from Nantucket, I floundered in trying to figure out a new direction. My success with writing for *Smart but Scattered Teens* reinforced a talent I felt I could tap, but my effort to transfer that to a job in publishing led nowhere. Back to college I went, but I found myself uninspired by the courses offered and dropped out. By all appearances, I had no successes to learn from, but some reflection proved otherwise.

Successful Strategies

• *When in doubt, take calculated risks.* Before agreeing to write the dialogues for *Smart but Scattered Teens*, I never thought writing for money was a possibility; maybe I had some raw talent, but all the evidence I'd seen said people who made it as writers were successful because they loved it and wrote all the time, and I'd never been all that prolific. But I knew the opportunity was rare, so I agreed without knowing what it would entail. I thought it would give me a big leg up, and it has, but not in the way I expected. Turns out when you're trying to get into the publishing business, being published isn't worth much compared to a degree or actual experience. But the book gave me some validation that people might respond and find what I say helpful or interesting. It gave me some much-needed money, and it lured me back to the idea of a career in social sciences. I think my lesson was that taking the leap to do this was worthwhile and not as much of a risk as it looked like beforehand. Professionally, in terms of my employment or career advancement, the book hasn't helped me very much yet, but, personally, the undertaking reoriented my path and taught me that some risks are worthwhile and necessary.

• *Always play to your strengths when you can.* My strengths are flexibility and emotional control. More generally, I also value my professional relationships and am respectful. Flexibility helped me take the leap into writing, landscaping, and working on a fishing boat. Even though none of these endeavors led to a career, they all cemented my ability to work hard and paid off in providing me with savings that kept me afloat between jobs. Not all the things I've done are integral to my career in an obvious way, but learning to work for and with almost anyone has frequently come in handy, and it makes me a more valuable employee because I'm versatile.

Jonas

Jonas succeeded in getting certified in cybersecurity, thanks in part to support from his mother for his weak time management, task initiation, and sustained attention skills. Based on the success he achieved with his mother's help, Jonas realized that he could use task initiation and time management apps with prompts he designed to take over these functions so he could meet both personal and work-related task deadlines. He supplemented these apps with tools that provided within-task prompts to ensure that he maintained on-task attention. We've referenced these tools in the Resources. When his manager at his current job offered him some additional work in this area and a modest pay increase, Jonas felt confident that he could manage the increased responsibility. He accepted the offer since he wanted the experience to test out his new skills, to improve his performance appraisals, and to add to his résumé if he looked for other positions. For now, he was content to build his hands-on knowledge and experience at his current job.

Successful Strategies

• *Keep goals modest.* For young adults who have worked hard at step-by-step SMART goals and reached a longer-term goal, as Jonas has, it can be tempting to get overconfident and speed things up. His mother is lobbying him to look for positions with more responsibility and pay, as well as to look at bachelor's degree programs in cybersecurity. Fortunately, using the techniques in Step 7, Jonas can visualize setting such a goal and quickly know he's not yet ready. Setting unrealistic goals is what led to his bouncing back from his first try at college. Jonas reminds his mother that the coursework required for a BS includes courses he has no interest in, and he doesn't want to repeat his previous experience of failure. Practicing implementation intentions, mental contrasting, and mental simulation while getting his certification has helped him develop his metacognition skills! He gently tells Marta that in the future, after he gets more experience, he might consider an associate's degree since he has met a number of the gen ed requirements that would be required. For many young adults with executive skills weaknesses, fairly modest SMART goals will remain the best way to get ahead in the long run.

Cheyenne

Cheyenne's executive skills weaknesses in goal-directed persistence and sustained attention undoubtedly factored into her dropping out of college, but it was her weakness in planning that really did her in. She had no clear idea where she was headed and therefore flitted somewhat randomly from one course to another without any vision of where she'd end up once she had a degree. Interestingly, many undergrads are in the same position until junior year, when something leads them to pick a certain major, whereupon they formulate a fuzzy picture of getting a job in "communications" or going to law school—only to realize upon graduating that they never really thought about whether this was what they really wanted to do. Cheyenne, in contrast, has reasonably strong metacognition, so she knows her strengths. But without a strong interest (real or fabricated), she had a hard time laying out a plan to get a degree at all. She was still having trouble figuring out a plan to identify a goal once she starting seeing all her friends move on. Fortunately, she knew she needed help, and she got it, from her father.

Successful Strategies

• *Seek and accept the help you need.* Many immobilized young adults have difficulty admitting that they need help from someone else, particularly a parent, to get moving. It takes time for some young adults to accept their weaknesses. Cheyenne's good metacognitive skills allowed her to admit she really couldn't plan and didn't know where to begin, so she was open to brainstorming with her father when he offered to help her. This is how she arrived at two possible career directions: marketing and military intelligence. Like many young adults, she didn't want her dad directing her life, but she knew he had good planning ability and she was happy to work with him on brainstorming possible directions. It became obvious that marketing jobs generally required a degree, and she found the job descriptions uninteresting, even though marketing in general seemed to satisfy her interests in psychology, work with people, and travel. Her dad wasn't thrilled with the idea of the military, but he knew better than to try to discourage her. Eventually Cheyenne decided on the Air National Guard, where her willingness to seek advice and direction continued to give her significant advantages.

• *Talk to others to open up your mind.* Young adults who are stuck at square one in identifying a goal often feel ashamed of not having any idea where to head. ("Everyone else seems to know what they want and where to go to get it. Why can't I?") This doesn't make them very likely to start a conversation (or even respond when others try to start one). And this reticence usually just keeps them stuck. The fact that Cheyenne was willing to brainstorm with her dad and then keep a dialogue going as she explored her options revealed ideas that might never have surfaced otherwise. When you're mentally stuck, trying to plan in your head is like trying to map out a route in a dark room, where you keep bumping into the same four walls, and the only input you get is the echo of your own voice.

Talking things out with her dad, she decided to meet with recruiters from the Army, Navy, Air Force, and Coast Guard. She was interested in the occupational options in the Army and Air Force but was wary of the 4-year commitment. But she did discover Special Investigations in the Air National Guard as an option and was intrigued by this since it seemed to fit well with her interests, the active-duty time commitment was acceptable and, if she liked the duties, she had the option of overseas deployment. Her state university offered a full tuition waiver for National Guard members, which meant that she could take courses related to this area and over time finish her degree without additional debt. And the idea of service to her country had particular appeal.

Cheyenne enlisted in the Air National Guard and began active duty training at the next available training cycle. By talking as openly as possible with her recruiter and reviewing the information he provided, she realized that there were career and pay advantages to completing her degree, so she has begun the necessary coursework. Her dad is proud that she has made this commitment and that she is motivated to complete school and has a direction. In addition, he feels that the service option she has chosen has made it less likely she will be in harm's way.

Once in the Air National Guard, Cheyenne sought advice from her commanding officer. Cheyenne had originally thought she was interested in intelligence operations in the Air Force. But she was told that there would be a delay in the training cycle for that specialty, which meant that she couldn't move ahead with her basic and occupational specialty training. In addition, she had recently deployed with her unit to assist communities with hurricane recovery and realized that she really enjoyed the work. Her unit's work had served both the physical and psychological needs of people in the community, and Cheyenne thought it fit well with her interest. Her commanding officer recognized the effort she had displayed while deployed, and they discussed whether this specialty, which was in high demand, might be a good fit for her. They also discussed the fact that her training would provide her with a readily transferable skill to civilian life, if that was a direction she wanted. Excited, and with her company commander's help, Cheyenne made a change in her military occupational specialty and after training settled in to her emergency management role in her unit.

Trafina

Trafina was living at home when we introduced her. She had just finished a job with City Year in Chicago and had moved back home and applied for some art teaching jobs. However, teacher certification was an issue, and beyond that her limited experience as a substitute art teacher led her to feel that this was not a career for her. From Trafina's perspective, the ideal situation would mimic her college experience, where she could go into a studio and create a work that she was interested in. Her executive skills weaknesses in flexibility and metacognition kept her from seeing other options that her art major might translate to, and she didn't see other skills that she might be able to bring to bear in some type of career.

People who experience weaknesses in flexibility and metacognition tend to keep coming back to the same types of solutions or options they had thought of in the first place. In Trafina's case, beyond the possibility of art teaching, which she did not find particularly appealing, she couldn't readily see other options and couldn't readily see next steps.

To get started, seeking help from another person who can offer a different perspective is the best option (as we noted with Cheyenne), as long as the person seeking help is open to suggestions from the helper. Trafina's mother suggested that by researching "careers for art majors" on the Internet Trafina might discover other possible careers in her interest area. Trafina was able to find some options she thought might be interesting, but she wasn't sure how to pursue them, so she returned to the career planning and placement office at her university, where her career counselor helped her reach the conclusion that graphic design might be an option for her. But without any education or experience in this specific area, she had only two options: go back to school or take an unpaid internship in a graphic design firm. Her mother had concerns that this would be her second year after graduation in a position that offered no financial support but realized it was a reasonable direction to pursue and something that might lead to a career for Trafina in a field she was interested in. On that basis, her parents agreed to support her through a full-time internship as long as it had some type of limited time commitment. Trafina was able to find, through career placement, a company that was comfortable with her doing a 6-month, unpaid, full-time internship and, with her parents' blessing Trafina took it.

Successful Strategies

• *Cultivate problem-solving skills to get around apparent dead ends.* Although weak in flexibility, Trafina has always enjoyed problem solving. It served her well in getting her bachelor's degree, and she called it into play (with some help from her mother in getting started) when she couldn't find a job that met her inflexible parameters and didn't know where else to turn. Graduate school would be too expensive, so where else could she get the experience she needed to see if she could make graphic arts a career goal? The internships were all unpaid, so how would she support herself when her parents had already helped her for a year after graduation? By talking to her mother, her career counselor, and others, and solving each individual problem step by step, Trafina overcame her inflexibility and is now halfway through her internship, where her supervisor and the people she works with have made her feel welcome. Her dependability, work ethic, and willingness to take on challenging projects have given them an appreciation of her skills. They've given her increasingly more responsibility, and Trafina has found she can use her art and technical skills and produce creative graphic solutions. The next problem to solve: how to convert the internship into a paid position in the graphic design business. While she doesn't have any definite commitment, her supervisor has hinted more than once that she has been a valuable addition to the firm and that they might be able to find a paying position for her.

Casey

Casey, 25, is living at home and has a steady income and reliable job as a teaching assistant in a public school that he likes well enough. His parents worry that he's too comfortable in a job that has no potential for moving up or out. At their instigation, he fills out the GTKMQ and is reminded that, besides liking to help people (an interest fulfilled at his current job), he used to be interested in health care. He recognizes that it's still an area of interest and has a lot more earning potential and job options, and he brings that up to his parents. They couldn't be more enthusiastic—in fact, they would have been wise to be a little less so. Immediately, they jumped into suggestions that he return to his "goal" of becoming a physician's assistant or a registered nurse as an alternative. The fact is that that "goal" was never very solid in Casey's mind, which is partially responsible (along with a fondness for the fun part of college life) for his having never finished his courses or received a degree. Casey knows from the Executive Skills Questionnaire that he has trouble with sustained attention and goal-directed persistence, but both weaknesses are situational. That is, he has learned that he is better able to maintain attention in a hands-on learning environment and in order to persist at a goal it needs to be motivating and achievable within a limited and foreseeable time frame. His teaching assistant job was motivating enough since he liked helping others, but now it feels like a dead end to both Casey and his parents. Knowing himself, however, led him to success on his journey toward independence.

Successful Strategies

• *Know how you learn best.* Casey has had several years to figure out that he has trouble with the usual academic routine but can thrive through experiential learning. He checks out options in health care that would make this possible and proposes to his parents that he start by becoming a certified nursing assistant and getting a job as a CNA, where he can learn more about the entire field of health care day by day and see how far he wants to go in this direction. They agree to support this route, especially knowing that there appear to be a fair number of jobs available and the pay is somewhat better than Casey makes as a teachers' aide. He completes the CNA training and is able to find a job on the pediatric floor of the local hospital since he likes working with children and his prior experience of working with children gives him a bit of a hiring advantage. After 6 months at this job with a variety of responsibilities, he is convinced that health care is the right field for him. The hospital that he's working at has an affiliation with the local community college that offers a licensed practical nursing (LPN) program and provides some tuition assistance as long as the recipient agrees to stay in the job for at least a year after he receives the degree. This option will also enable him to continue working part time and to acquire his practical experience in doing so. He finishes his LPN training and accepts an LPN position at his hospital with a significant increase in pay.

Casey is also learning through his current experience that he would like to progress further, and while working as an LPN he looks into programs where he can complete his training to become a registered nurse (RN) and decides to pursue this goal. While his eventual goal of being an RN could have taken a more direct path, the path that Casey has chosen is a measured approach that takes advantage of his hands-on learning style, allows him to get experience at a variety of different levels in the field, and quite possibly provides a level of training and experience that a traditional RN program might not give him. In addition, his approach allows him to make good use of financial resources so that across his training he is able to increase his financial self-sufficiency.

• *Take one step at a time to correct your course as needed and stay on track.* Again, parents (and some young adults) often want to catapult their son or daughter onto the path toward a distant goal. The final destination seems so far off that many young adults get discouraged right away. Or they become anxious about all the points along the way where they might "fail" and get frozen or start to stumble. Casey's metacognition is pretty well developed at the age of 25, and he feels strongly about learning through experience what he wants, can do, and enjoys, and moving forward in individual steps instead of committing to a physician's assistant or RN job right from the start. This approach allows him to learn at every step and make course corrections in his plan whenever needed. When he eventually does become an RN, this thoughtful approach will make him one of the most highly valued pediatric nurses in the hospital.

Gina, Dion, Jayden, James

Gina, introduced in Step 3, has also been developing a greater degree of metacognition over time. At first she mistook her ability to soothe injured children for an inclination toward the health care field, a perception helped along by the fact that her mother is a nurse. Now, there certainly isn't anything wrong with wanting to pursue the same career as a parent. The important metacognitive point is that Gina be *aware* that her mother's career might be exerting some influence on her decision making. There are known and unknown factors affecting all of the decisions we make. Our job as good metacognicians is to identify and gauge them; engaging in this process systematically and repeatedly will over time increase our ability to understand our skills, appraise situations, and make sound decisions.

As with Gina, part of this process is gathering information and deliberating on it in light of personal preferences. When people are motivated to solve their problems, it often seems like they move to short, staccato decisions that *feel* efficient, demonstrative, and momentous. But choosing entire career paths based on their titles and apparent fit is a time waster if it means languishing for an extended time in the wrong place until washing out and beginning the cycle again.

Both Gina and Dion, our would-be vet, recognized their skills and preferences, but initially opted for careers without full awareness of whether their skills were a match for the career-path demands. Once exposed to these demands, both realized the skill–demand mismatch and shifted to related careers where skills, preferences, and demands were a fit. Both were able to bring their metacognitive skills to bear in the context of newly acquired information.

For Jayden, our bachelor's degree English major with a penchant for text analysis and writing, and James, our bachelor's degree English major and would-be lawyer, the path was more circuitous and somewhat serendipitous. Jayden, for example, had a bit of a sunk cost fallacy going on; he had a liberal arts BA and a belief that to maximize it teaching might need to be the path, but for him this was a preference nonstarter. For James, the demand path for a legal degree eliminated this career notion. Jayden, pressed for money, didn't consider technical writing as a possible fit for his skills and preferences. We can't necessarily fault his metacognitive skills for this; he knew what he liked and was skilled in. More likely it was some weakness in flexibility in thinking about writing careers. But the necessity for earning money along with the serendipity and metacognitive skills of a friend and an interviewer, who saw his potential fit, resulted in a career match.

James did what a lot of college grads with a liberal arts BA do—he landed a job that required a BA but no other specific skill set that paid the bills. His performance problems were a testament to the misfit. He used his metacognitive self-appraisal skill to reject his parents' career suggestions. While on the face of it, his choice of construction seems driven by monetary necessity combined with the opportunity of a friend's connection, in fact it is more informed than that. He reviews his history and knows what he likes. While he views the job as a "placeholder" for now, there are factors that suggest it may turn out otherwise. He chose the job based on his preferences; a known, proven skill set; and excitement about the work. Construction may not turn out to be his life-long career, but it is the best fit he's had since graduating and he is arguably well on his way to independent living.

The real world contains a lot more forks and twists in the road forward, and "where you start isn't where you'll end up" is as likely the rule as the exception. So we encourage all young adults to think of their skills and preferences and how they match with the path chosen. The effort and hurdles aren't trivial, but understanding where you're motivated to go is the crux.

Epilogue

This epilogue is late.

And written in eerily similar circumstances to the Introduction you read 200-odd pages ago. Again I am sitting in the living room on the second floor of an apartment in November, peeking over the top of the same laptop screen to see cars, canted old brick buildings, and wind pulling off yellow leaves and stirring them into shaded corners. My favorite football podcast is in the background, and I can see a skim layer of pollen on the lit portions of the sill. And I am late on a third deadline.

Hypothetically, I need to finish a draft in less than 45 minutes in order to shower, ice a sore elbow, change laundry over, clean my car, and leave at 1:00 P.M. and be at my girlfriend's around 3:00.

Maybe the difference, between then and now, is that I will make it.

I am still in school, still working to motivate myself for work that doesn't interest me, still asking for extensions after the fact.

But now it is graduate school, in a field I've committed to. I don't know about passion, I don't think I know what other people are feeling when they use that term. But it is a theory and a practice of studying and trying to improve human behavior that I am obsessed with and the type of job I've stayed in the longest.

I moved home after two and a half years of living in St. Louis. My relationship failed, but I learned from it. I failed, again, at school, and learned from that. I was good at my job, and learned that there was something about it that intrigued me. I drove to St. Louis by myself, and when I came back my dad drove with me. I was very grateful for this.

Back home, I found new friends and old ones. I got it together and finished school, and not without a sort of macabre, foreboding sense of humor I applied for grad school before I got my diploma. It was difficult, to put it mildly, to think that getting back in the water before I was even dry was a good idea, but the work that drove me drives my school now in a way that it didn't before.

And there is a new relationship, a different kind of relationship that maybe comes with time or age or experience. I don't know, I think what I notice is not only the other person making me happy, but deriving happiness from a commitment that sometimes means making trade-offs, but that delivers a longer-term satisfaction with doing what one feels like the right thing is.

Applied behavior analysis (ABA), the discipline I work with and learn about, is used most often with children with autism and intellectual disabilities. It deals with the impact of events on human behavior and using data about the effect on behavior to make positive changes for individuals and communities. It has gained prominence in use for individuals with these disorders, although it is also gaining popularity for workplace and business applications.

ABA relies on a research method called single-subject design (only one person in the study) in order to precisely document how an event changes behavior and to make future predictions from these data. Since entering this field, I've started to see my life and behavior as a 30-year single-subject design experiment. It isn't always well controlled or unbiased or all that rigorous, but I have a mountain of data to pore over continuously, trying to figure out why I do what I do, and how I might do it differently, better, the next time.

When I left St. Louis, it became clear I'd need to rent a trailer, to account for the lost storage space in the front seat that would now be displaced by my dad. Instead my dad convinced me to go through my stuff again, and I left a lot behind at the Goodwill and in the dumpster next to my building. It was hard, and I later remember thinking how silly it was that it was hard, because I threw away even more once I got home and unpacked. It was shed it or accept the price it'd extract to keep it. Like old and accumulating goods, past experiences extract a price and act like an anchor. Shedding things is a part of life. I haven't, can't, and don't want to erase the past, but I've learned there is merit in putting it behind me and putting a fresh foot forward. My mom one time gave me a refrigerator magnet with a Ralph Waldo Emerson quote that begins "Finish each day and be done with it, you've done what you could. . . ." I look at it and think of it a lot because I think the message is spot-on. There are a lot of them, but each day is important. You can't (and shouldn't) forget or rewrite the past, but you can move on from it, and time is your ally if you spend it looking more at the new days and less at the old ones. My hope for anyone reading this book, young adult or parent, is that it helps you do just that—take a look at the past, get the information from it that will serve you best, and move on.

COLIN GUARE, 2017

Appendix

··

Getting Help with Independent Living

Throughout this book we've focused on strategies that young adults and parents can collaborate on to help young adults reach independence. In this Appendix we offer resources that will help young adults approaching independence take on the tasks of daily living that parents have been completely doing for them or helping them manage. Naturally, you'll continue to provide advice and recommendations, but mainly when the young adult requests it or in the form of some modeling and training when the young adult has no experience with the task at all. This transition from parents to community-based resources is a very concrete marker for the young adult's independence from the parent's former "official role" as both advice giver and decider. All adults use community and online resources to help them with practical necessities, from providing themselves with food and shelter to getting a job and managing money, and all young adults need to be able to find reliable expert advice and service tailored to their needs. Does your young adult know how to perform the following tasks?

- How and where to grocery shop
- How to find and apply for a job
- How to locate and cost out an apartment
- How to use banking and money services, including credit cards, checking accounts, debit cards, and ATMs
- How to buy health insurance
- How to access medical and dental care
- How to buy a car
- How to register, obtain a title for, and have the car inspected
- How to buy auto insurance
- How to manage car repairs, car maintenance, and breakdowns

If you and your young adult are concerned about independent living skills beyond those involved in these tasks, a form to use for a comprehensive assessment of skill areas is available from *www.crporegon.org* Paste this URL into your browser. When you reach the site, using their search box, put in Ansell-Casey Life Skills Assessment. That will provide you with a link to the assessment tool. If you are interested in a shorter, less formal list of skills for young adults, paste the following link into your browser: *https://patch.com/connecticut/darien/bp--before-they-leave-home-de7d761c.*

As you'll see next, for some of the areas in the list of tasks parents may still play a significant role. But when the young adult begins to shift to relying on outside sources for help with the tasks of adult life, both the young adult and the parent benefit in several ways:

- The young adult has a chance to learn how to evaluate different sources of information and services in a way that takes into consideration her resources and priorities (e.g., cost, location).

- Outside resources offer current, "real-world" advice and expertise that exceeds the breadth and depth that most parents could offer.

- As a result, when the young adult turns to outside resources parents are absolved of the temptations to resume a "I know what is best for you" hierarchical parent role.

- This in turn can help to diffuse any conflicts that may crop up in the relationship between young adult and parent, especially those precipitated by the parent trying to direct the young adult.

- Finally, by searching for and utilizing these various resources in the community, the young adult gradually builds a support network that he can expand and turn to across his lifespan.

Since our objective throughout this book has been facilitating independence in young adults, we thought it best to get their opinions. So we sampled a group of millennials (those born from 1980 on) to hear their thoughts about how they would search for and access these community resources. Our sample ranged from young adults living at home and un- or underemployed to those living on their own who had a job. Their educational levels ranged from high school diploma or GED to college graduate. They all shared the common feature of continuing to rely on some degree of parental support, usually financial.

With the exception of a few services, which we'll note, the consensus across the sample was that they would begin their search using the Internet. Their search options ranged from a direct search of the category (e.g., apartments, insurance) to querying friends and contacts on social media such as Facebook and LinkedIn. We will briefly discuss by category each of the identified services and include the Internet sources that they suggested as well as those that we are familiar with that they might not have noted.

Not all young adults will need these resources, so young adults and parents can pick and choose those that seem valuable. For each category below, we'll note how parents can use their experience with the tasks to add value to the resources identified by the young adult—wherever the young adult is open to that.

Grocery Shopping

This an experience-based skill where Internet information has little or no application. For young adults who have always lived at home (or at college, on a meal plan) or will be buying food on a limited budget for the first time, a little training using an apprenticeship model can be helpful. Practical as well as executive skills (planning and organization, task initiation, sustained attention and response inhibition, and flexibility) come into play in meal planning and identifying needed cleaning products, bathroom supplies, and all of the staples that are part of meal planning, such as condiments and dairy products.

Here are some steps the young adult can take to get started on a shopping list:

1. Review typical family meals and list the foods that go into them for a regular week.
2. Look through refrigerators, cabinets, or pantries to list the foods routinely consumed, including snacks.
3. Review with parents (who can then ask open-ended questions about missing items).
4. Add brand names (most people shop for specific brands) and be sure to note size.
5. Once the list is reasonably complete, you can consider organizing it by the typical supermarket department or aisle.

Now for the shopping:

1. Establish that the young adult is generally familiar with the scheme of grocery stores (the produce department, the frozen-food aisle, the butcher case, etc.).
2. If the family favors a certain store, discuss why.
3. Discuss any price considerations after checking out: Did you decide to skip certain items on this trip because the price had gone up and they're not essential for a meal? Did you decide to try a different brand than usual because of a special deal?
4. To teach comparison shopping, consider taking a small sample from the grocery list and buying these items in a subsequent trip at a different store to

compare prices and demonstrate that the selection per store as well as price of item can vary significantly.

Over time, the objective is for the young adult to plan selected meals, independently make lists of the items needed to prepare the meal, and independently shop for them.

Introducing Banking Services, Credit and Debit Cards, ATMs, and Other Credit Issues

Young adults who as children have shopped with their parents in any fashion will have seen their parents use credit and debit cards, and most parents have talked to their children about the subject. As parents of young adults and as a young adult we have experienced the benefits and risks of credit and debit cards and the importance of understanding basic financial management as it relates to these topics. The overriding concern for all adults, young adults included, is the ease with which you can spend more than you can afford. Credit cards, particularly in the hands of young adults who are inexperienced, can make that overspending relatively easy. The resulting problems, after the fact, include barriers to apartment rentals, car purchases, and jobs, just to name a few of the more serious results. In addition, it means being subjected to a barrage of telephone calls, e-mails, and letters regarding late payments.

For young adults who are new to the world of credit and debit cards and the associated risks we prefer options that involve some type of spending limits.

- Debit cards, both prepaid and those tied to a bank checking account. The problem with debit cards tied to bank checking accounts is the issue of overdraft fees. In addition, debit cards do not help to build credit scores and a good credit history.

- A "secured credit card," which requires making a refundable deposit as collateral to secure the account, analogous to any type of security deposit.

To explore these options and others, check out the sources we have found most helpful at the time this book is being written.

- Credit Karma (*www.creditkarma.com*), a free credit and financial platform on the Internet and on mobile platforms such as IOS and Android.

- NERDWALLET (*www.nerdwallet.com*), a free tool that offers a wide range of information about debit and credit cards, bank overdrafts on debit cards and checking cards, and a range of other financial products.

- Banking specialists who are available to discuss this information. They have a wealth of information, and if your children are living at home or are living somewhere in the same geographic area, oftentimes they will utilize the same resources.

Finding Health Insurance

With the advent of the Affordable Care Act (ACA, or "Obamacare"), significant changes occurred for young adults. The health insurance market and its laws were in a state of flux as we wrote this book. As of late 2017, these were (in broad strokes) the options available to many young adults:

- Young adults 26 or under can be covered by their parents' health insurance. For details or conditions of this coverage, go to *www.healthcare.gov/young-adults/children-under-26*.

- Health insurance through the ACA (*www.healthcare.gov*). Unfortunately, the information available online is very complicated, so we recommend visiting an independent insurance agent; see, for example, the Mutual Benefit Group's "7 Reasons to Choose an Independent Agent" at *https://tinyurl.com/ybqqloe9*.

- Health insurance through their college or university if enrolled.

- Employer-sponsored health plans for those who are employed (with different costs depending on the plan selected).

> Many young adults, either through deliberate choice or lack of information, do not have health insurance. They should understand that parents will do everything in their power to ensure the young adult's recovery from illness or injury, which may mean accruing crushing debt. Thus, by not having insurance, young adults may unintentionally put their parents at significant financial risk.

Finding and Accessing Medical and Dental Care

Of course, the type of insurance chosen often determines which medical and dental practitioners and providers the young adult can see, what services are covered, and to what extent. Since primary care physicians (PCP) are the gatekeepers for health care, locating a PCP who is covered by insurance is key for the young adult. Insurance companies provide names of physicians in their networks, and increasingly one can find ratings available for doctors (e.g., we've found *www.vitals.com* to be helpful). The primary task for young adults who are new to their own health care is to schedule their own health care appointments, which ideally started when they were teenagers.

Beyond setting up appointments, the most critical aspect for young adults (all adults in fact) is making good use of the physicians' knowledge and advocating for themselves. Again, the best source of this information for adults is the Internet. Using Google and searching the question "What questions to ask your physician?" yields a variety of resources, including trustworthy sources of information about symptoms. If young adults are not comfortable with this approach, it can be helpful for parents to discuss with them what their questions/concerns might be. In the case of young adults who are very reluctant or anxious, accompanying them to the first visit and prompting or modeling for them the questions to ask can be very helpful and an important step in the hand-off to the doctor.

Finding a Job

Many young adults will have part- or full-time job experience from work during their teen years. Job search strategies that they used then may still apply, depending on the types of jobs they're looking for. Let's consider young adults with or without postsecondary education who are living at home and either not working or working part time. For them, the first objective is to get a job or to work more hours.

If the point is to generate some income and not develop a career track at this point, the best resources are:

- Networking with friends who are currently working and may know of jobs with their own employer or other related employment resources
- Craigslist and online newspaper job postings
- Parents as networking resources. Since I worked with a number of different schools and agencies, I was often aware of their job postings, and in some cases Colin subsequently went to work in these agencies because he had an interest and the skill set.

For young adults searching for jobs beyond entry-level employment, the following web-based resources provide information about job search strategies.

- *www.jobdiagnosis.com/blog/attention-young-adults-job-search-strategies-for-millennials*
- *www.monster.com/career-advice/article*

For a list of the best job search websites:

- *www.roberthalf.com/job-seekers/career-center/job-hunting-tips/10-best-job-search-websites*. While the lists vary from source to source, there is general agreement about the websites that are thought to be best.

For individuals who are in college or have earned a degree:

- Career planning and placement offices/resources of colleges and universities are a valuable source for jobs, internships, and assessments for career preferences.

For young adults who do not have access to these resources, the following links provide a comprehensive list of job and career resources, including self-assessment tools, occupational and salary information, employment trends, and job search assistance. Both offer excellent job and career development resources.

- *www.ncda.org/aws/NCDA/pt/sp/resources*
- *http://youth.gov/youth-topics/youth-employment/career-exploration-and-skill-development*

Finally, many if not most states offer a host of state-sponsored employment services and resources. Some adults will be familiar with these services if they have ever received unemployment compensation. These employment offices are a rich source of job postings, career counseling, and vocational/career evaluation services that can help young adults identify interest areas and potential matching jobs. In our experience, this is a generally unfamiliar and underutilized resource that can provide hands-on, informed, professional help to young adults that is free of charge. The following website provides information about these resources in states across the country.

- *https://usnlx.com/state-workforce-agencies.asp*

Locating and Costing Out an Apartment

The young adults that we sampled identified the following three websites as resources that they have used to start their apartment search:

- *www.zillow.com/rent*
- *www.apartments.com*
- *www.craigslist.org/about/sites*

The consensus of our sample was that even young adults who are currently not in the market to rent should go through the search process for practice. In this case the young adult identifies a couple of different apartments within a designated price range and then via e-mail or telephone contacts the apartment source to assess if the apartment is still available and if so, to arrange a time to see it. For young adults with limited or no experience in apartment searches, friends or parents can work with them on a list of questions about the apartment. Beyond the actual rent, this includes upfront costs such as security deposits, a-month-in-advance deposit, length of the lease, cost to break the lease, cost of utilities and what is included, parking, and restrictions (pets, parties, etc.). Gathering this information helps the young adult plan the costs that will need to be considered, whether roommates will be necessary, and the types of conditions the young adult is likely to be living in.

Transportation: Investigating the Options

Young adults living in large urban areas with good access to public transportation may use that as their primary means of getting around to jobs, stores, and other resources in the community. For many young adults, however, transportation will involve a car and eventually car ownership, since access to family vehicles is likely to be time limited. Therefore, most young adults should know at least the basics of car buying even if they aren't in the market right now. Experience with the process in a hands-on fashion enhances their knowledge base and skills, including planning, task initiation, and response inhibition. Two resources, taken together, offer important information about price and reliability for both new and used cars:

- The Kelley Blue Book (*www.kbb.com*), which allows the young adult to put in all of the particulars about a car (age, mileage, model type, etc.), and provides a reliable range of the car's value tied to the area in which you search.
- CARFAX (*www.carfax.com*), which provides information about the repair history of the car based on the specific automobile identification number. A detailed report involves some expense, but the expense is small when considering that the purchase price of even a used car can involve thousands of dollars. Again, even if the young adult is not currently searching for a car, this experience allows her to engage in the fantasy of having a car and going through the process of investigating the car search and buying process.

We have done this with our two young adults, including visiting dealerships and people with private sales and test driving the vehicles. For future reference, it is important to investigate how the car will be purchased, particularly if some type of financing is involved. This information is readily accessed online by looking at the banks or financial intuitions that the young adult and/or parent does business with. Young adults also need information about automobile registration and titles, which are required across all states.

The next step, if a vehicle is to be purchased, is investigating the availability and cost of auto insurance. At the current time, auto insurance is optional in only one state, New Hampshire, where the authors reside. *Regardless of where young adults reside, even if automobile insurance is not mandatory, it is essential.* While even relatively minor car repairs related to an accident can be prohibitively expensive, the cost and associated stress pale in comparison to liabilities associated with personal injury claims. A cautionary tale from our own family's experience: In her mid-20s, our daughter was in a minor accident. Soon after the accident, she was served a subpoena for a court appearance by a deputy sheriff at 6:30 in the morning. The subpoena involved a civil liability claim involving purported personal injury claimed by an occupant of the other car. While our daughter was judged to be at no fault and the police did not file a report due to the minor nature of the accident, the subpoena (her first) was quite real and created a great deal of stress for her, including over her lack of financial resources. Fortunately, at the time of the accident she had her own auto insurance, and the insurance company stepped in immediately to help her with the claim and hired an attorney to defend her and the company from liability. *The need for quality automobile insurance coverage cannot be underestimated.*

Where does one find good affordable coverage for young adults? By searching "best automobile insurance for young adults" on the Internet, we were able to readily identify a group of companies that were well rated for their affordability and quality, and that offer at least estimated quotes online. Since obtaining these quotes involves no commitment from young adults, we recommend that they use information on the car that they are interested in, if even only hypothetically. And this should include comparison shopping among different companies to get estimated rates based on the type of vehicle, driver characteristics, and the zip code in which the young adult lives. This will provide the young adult a real practice opportunity that she would benefit from having when she does decide to buy an automobile.

Finally, there is the issue of auto maintenance and repairs. If the young adult does not currently have a car and uses a family auto, take him to the family's mechanic or car dealership. Having witnessed the process of getting a car serviced a few times, the next step is to have the young adult take the car for repairs or maintenance himself. If the problem needing attention is not readily identified, the young adult and parent can discuss this issue and come up with questions for the mechanic. For a young adult who has his own auto and is living in a location different from the parent, networking with friends and peers at work regarding available and reliable repair services can be quite effective. If peers have been in the area for a while, then you benefit from their local knowledge and experience, especially if you share their current socioeconomic status. If parents use automotive associations such as AAA, we highly recommend family memberships that include the young adult. The cost tends to be within reason, and since young adults, particularly if they're starting out, tend to be driving older car models with higher mileage, the availability of fast and reliable road service is a significant "peace of mind" option for both the young adult and parents.

Miscellaneous Resources

Coaching Resources Offering Executive Skills Informed Coaching

www.mythrive.net/_pages/programs/executive_function.htm

The Thrive Center is located in Columbia, MD. Thrive offers a number of different coaching options as well as a transition program for young adults who are struggling to launch. The program is provided in the context of a peer cohort. The center also offers comprehensive psychological services.

www.drhallowell.com/the-hallowell-centers/evaluative-and-ongoing-services

The Hallowell Centers have locations on the East and West coasts of the United States. The centers were founded by Dr. Edward (Ned) Hallowell, a psychiatrist and world-renowned expert in ADHD. The centers provide a number of different executive skills–informed coaching options for children, adolescents, and adults—with the option of online coaching—as well as comprehensive psychological services.

www.advancela.org/one-on-one%20coaching

Advance LA is located in metropolitan Los Angeles and is a program within The Help Group, the largest and most comprehensive nonprofit in the United States providing services to children through adults with special needs. Advance LA specializes in the transitional issues of adolescents and young adults. They offer a range of different coaching options, including executive function skills coaching as well as a variety of other programs to facilitate successful transitions to more self-sufficient living. Advance LA and The Help Group also provide an extensive range of psychological services.

www.beyondbooksmart.com/academic-coaching-college-executive-functioning-strategies

Beyond Book Smart is a company with locations in the Boston area and many parts of the country. The company specializes in providing executive function coaching in academic areas for children, adolescents, and adults. They have highly trained staff, and in our opinion are an excellent resource for executive skills–informed coaching for individuals in academic settings. They now offer extensive online coaching options.

www.yellincenter.com/coaching-and-consultation-for-executive-functioning.html

We are not familiar with this coaching program in New York City, but Dr. Edelstein's training and qualifications and her association with the Yellin Center suggest that it is a quality service for executive skills–informed academic coaching.

www.chadd.org/Understanding-ADHD/About-ADHD/Treatment-of-ADHD/
Complementary-and-Other-Interventions/Coaching.aspx

CHADD (Children and Adults with Attention Deficit/Hyperactivity Disorder): The National Resource for ADHD has excellent guidelines about coaching. Not all young adults have weaknesses in executive skills, but children and adults with ADHD typically have a range of executive skills weaknesses. Hence, many coaches in this area will be familiar with executive skills and effective intervention strategies for coach.

Resources for Psychological Issues

Each of the following websites provides resources for parents and young adults regarding the psychological issues that can arise in emerging adulthood. In addition to describing these issues, these websites provide access to additional resources for consultation and intervention for these issues.

www.rtor.org/emerging-adults
www.goodtherapy.org/learn-about-therapy/issues/young-adults
www.nami.org/Find-Support/Teens-and-Young-Adults

Cell Phones

If parents have the resources, family plans are often less expensive than each individual in the family having a separate plan. In our family, my wife and I share a plan with our daughter and son. When they have the resources, we expect that each will pay for part of the basic service and we limit the data options. If they exceed the monthly data allowed, they are responsible for the charges. In return for this expense, we expect that, as needed, they will return texts or calls from us when we need information from them within a reasonable time frame, which is typically 4 hours unless we need an immediate response. They are each responsible for their own phone choice, repairs, and replacement cost, although if my wife or I have upgrades available, if we don't need them, we make them available to our children.

Education Loans

As we said previously, the young adult should have some "skin in the game." If possible, young adults should be responsible for researching and arranging their own financial assistance. College financial aid offices are the among the best sources of information since they have an interest in seeing students enroll. In some cases, young adults will not be able to secure loans without someone to cosign, and this is most likely to be the parent. If you choose to do this for your young adult, we strongly recommend that, if possible, you do this for only a semester at a time. In addition, we recommend that you make your continued support contingent on achievement of specific grades that are decided in advance. We also recommend that young adults who have had past difficulties in school seek out the least-expensive school option, which will typically be the community college system.

Resources

The following print and Internet resources, plus smart phone apps, focus mainly on executive skills. For apps and other resources that help young adults with the tasks of daily living, see the Appendix.

Books

Aladina, S. (2015). *The mindful way through stress: The proven 8-week path to health, happiness, and well-being.* New York: Guilford Press.

Not all of us have the opportunity or the resources to go to a mindfulness retreat to learn this kind of meditation. This book gives you the chance to learn mindfulness meditation at home, following an 8-week step-by-step program that is actually two programs: a mini-course for people for whom time is at a premium and a more complete program for those who have the time to delve more deeply into the practice. The book also comes with downloadable meditations.

Barkley, R. A. (1997). *ADHD and the nature of self-control.* New York: Guilford Press.

Barkley, R. A. (2012). *Executive functions: What they are, how they work, and why they evolved.* New York: Guilford Press.

While technical, both these books help the reader understand ADHD as well as executive skills. Written by a leading expert on ADHD, Barkley makes the case in the first book that ADHD is, at base, a disorder involving executive skills, while in the second he offers a comprehensive theory of executive skills, combining neuropsychological and evolutionary research.

Barkley, R. A. (2010). *Taking charge of adult ADHD*. New York: Guilford Press.

Barkley converts his vast knowledge of ADHD into practical, everyday strategies for adults to address the executive skill and daily living issues associated with ADHD.

Baumeister, R. F., & Tierney, J. (2011). *Willpower: Rediscovering the greatest human strength*. New York: Penguin Books.

Written by a leading researcher on the topic, this book summarizes the research on self-control and gives the reader not only a window into how psychologists understand self-control but how they identify effective strategies for improving this critical skill.

Begley, S. (2007). *Train your mind, change your brain: How a new science reveals our extraordinary potential to transform ourselves*. New York: Ballantine Books.

The author, a well-known science writer, reports on how cutting-edge science and the ancient wisdom of Buddhism have come together to reveal that, contrary to popular belief, we have the power to literally change our brains by changing our minds. An accessible book that helps the reader understand neuroplasticity.

Brier, N. M. (2015). *Enhancing self-control in adolescents: Treatment strategies derived from psychological science*. New York: Routledge.

While this book focuses on adolescents, Brier provides excellent explanations and examples of motivational interviewing, implementation intentions with mental contrasting, and mental simulation that parents and young adults could easily adapt for their own use. It is also an excellent resource for coaches and cognitive-behavioral therapists for use with their clients.

Davidson, R. J., & Begley, S. (2012). *The emotional life of your brain: How its unique patterns affect the way you think, feel, and live—and how you can change them*. New York: Hudson Street Press.

In this book, Begley combines forces with Richard Davidson, a pioneering neuroscientist, focusing on the neurological basis of emotions. They describe six distinctive brain patterns associated with different emotional styles, referencing research from Dr. Davidson's laboratory to support their framework.

Dawson, P., & Guare, R. (2016). *The smart but scattered guide to success: How to use your brain's executive skills to keep up, stay calm, and get organized at work and at home*. New York: Guilford Press.

Continuing their work on strategies to improve executive skills, Dawson and Guare have written a self-help book containing a host of detailed plans to enhance these skills. Parents and young adults can use this book to add to their understanding of problem-solving approaches.

Gawande, A. (2009). *The checklist manifesto: How to get things right.* New York: Holt.

Atul Gawande is a surgeon who writes about medical issues for a lay audience. In this book, he describes how checklists can be a vital tool to preserve the health and safety of consumers (patients and airline passengers, among others). After reading this book, you may decide that checklists are the survival tool for life in the 21st century.

Hallowell, E. M., & Ratey, J. J. (2011). *Driven to distraction, revised edition.* New York: Anchor.

A classic, updated, in the field of adult ADHD, offering a thorough explanation, coping strategies, and the range of treatment options available.

Harris, D. (2014). *10% happier: How I tamed the voice in my head, reduced stress without losing my edge, and found self-help that actually works—a true story.* New York: HarperCollins.

If you're intrigued with the idea of mindfulness meditation but are skeptical all the same, read this book. Dan Harris, an ABC correspondent, writes a compelling first sentence: "According to the Nielsen ratings data, 5.019 million people saw me lose my mind." After having a panic attack on national television, Dan went searching for help. He looked to neuroscience, religion, and self-help gurus for a path forward, and ended up with mindfulness meditation. A fun book that packs a lot of information between the covers.

Konstam, V. (2015). *Emerging and young adulthood: Multiple perspectives, diverse narratives* (2nd ed.). New York: Springer.

This book is written as a resource for clinicians and researchers. Konstam sees emerging adulthood as the period from 18 to 30 years of age, and her research, gathered from a wide range of sources, provides a good summary of current thinking in the field. Of interest to clinicians as well as perhaps parents and young adults are the variety of narratives she collects from young adults, parents, and employers.

Levitan, D. J. (2014). *The organized mind: Thinking straight in the age of information overload.* New York: Dutton.

Keeping track of things and staying organized in a world filled to capacity with information is not easy. Other books in this resource list address response inhibition. This one looks at organization, working memory, and time management. As with other books on our list, this one combines neuroscience with practical suggestions.

Maurer, R. (2014). *One small step can change your life: The Kaizan way.* New York: Workman.

We can't say enough about this book. We've been believers for a long time in a "baby steps" approach to behavior change. This book not only shows why that's the way to go but provides compelling stories about how it works.

Mischel, W. (2014). *The marshmallow test: Mastering self-control.* New York: Little, Brown.

The marshmallow test is the best-known research study showing the impact of self-control on behavior, starting in preschool and continuing throughout life. Mischel makes the case that this is a skill that can be modified through the use of cognitive strategies, and the book provides ample examples of this.

Naar-King, S., & Suarez, M. (2011). *Motivational interviewing with adolescents and young adults.* New York: Guilford Press.

While technical in its approach and targeted to coaches and clinicians, this book provides a thorough explanation and examples of motivational interviewing with young adults. The authors make a strong case that motivation for a lasting change in behavior must begin with the young adult and cannot originate with parents, coaches, or clinicians.

Oettigen, G. (2014). *Rethinking positive thinking: Inside the new science of motivation.* New York, NY: Current.

This book is an excellent layperson's introduction to the work of Oettigen and her colleagues on implementation intentions with mental contrasting and her goal attainment strategy of WOOP (wish, outcome, obstacle, plan), a strategy that she and her colleagues have validated in a variety of research and clinical studies. (See her app, **WOOP,** on page 275.)

Perry, J. (2012). *The art of procrastination: A guide to effective dawdling, lollygagging and postponing.* New York: Workman.

This is a light-hearted take on procrastination written by an emeritus professor of philosophy at Stanford University. He describes a productive way that procrastinators can become more effective in managing this bad habit by using a method he calls "productive procrastination."

Weyandt, L,. & DuPaul, G. (2013). *College students with ADHD: Current issues and future directions.* New York: Springer.

Although this book is intended for professionals, parents may be interested in the data on how ADHD persists beyond adolescence. A chapter on ADHD in middle and high school also includes some helpful information on making the transition from secondary school to college.

Magazines, Periodicals, and Newsletters

ADDitude

This magazine is chock-full of strategies and supports for people with weak executive skills. Even if you don't have ADHD, you will find this magazine helpful (a recent issue had a cover story entitled "47 Must-Have Apps—Get Your Life in Order Now"). They also have a useful website: *www.ADDitudeMagazine.com.*

ATTENTION!

This is the official publication of Children and Adults with Attention-Deficit/Hyperactivity Disorder (CHADD). It also offers practical strategies and resources for managing the symptoms of ADHD. CHADD's website is *www.chadd.org*.

Brain in the News

This is a free monthly newsletter published by the Dana Foundation, whose mission is to advance brain research and educate the public responsibly about advances in brain science. Check out their website (which also provides links to other great websites) and sign up for their newsletter at *www.dana.org*.

Scientific American Mind

This is a bimonthly popular science magazine that translates research on the brain and cognitive science into accessible, readable articles on topics that readers can apply to their everyday lives. Their website is *www.scientificamerican.com/magazine/mind*.

Useful Websites

In addition to the resources just listed, here are some helpful and informative websites:

Headspace
www.headspace.com

There are lots of resources available for people who want to pursue mindfulness meditation. This is one of our favorites—developed by Andy Puddicombe, a former Buddhist priest based in the United Kingdom. It offers a series of guided meditations using a number of different techniques. There's a subscription involved, but the first 10 days are free, so check it out first. As we've explored mindfulness resources, we've discovered that the voice that guides you through a meditation practice is really important. We happen to like Andy's voice, but listen for yourself.

ISHA Foundation
www.ishafoundation.org

Another website that provides guided meditations as well as videos about meditation. This site offers free materials.

Medscape
www.medscape.com

This is another website that features health news—particularly useful to track research on aging as well as current practice in treating mental health issues such as ADHD, anxiety, and depression.

The MGH Clay Center for Healthy Young Minds

www.mghclaycenter.org

This website, while not exclusively focused on young adults, contains a variety of information and resources for parents and young adults about developmental features, typical struggles, and resources to help.

Science Daily

www.sciencedaily.com

This website features breaking news about the latest discoveries in health and science from major news services and leading universities, scientific journals, and resource organizations. Sign up for one of their newsletters and it will be sent to your inbox.

Smart Phone Apps and Other Technology for Executive Skills

Throughout this book, we've mentioned the use of smart phones to assist with various aspects of executive skills. In addition to smart phone apps that we have mentioned in the text, we offer the following as aids. For convenience, we have grouped them according to the executive skills for which they seem most applicable. In some cases, an app may be relevant to more than one executive skill. Not all executive skills are represented here because at the time of this writing we could not find apps that we considered directly relevant. By the time you read this book, however, new and better apps may be available that you can find by conducting an Internet search.

Response Inhibition/Sustained Attention

- **StayFocusd.** This app works on Google Chrome and allows you to limit the amount of time you spend on "time-wasting websites." You determine how much time per day you'll allow yourself to go to those websites, and when the time is up, your access to them is denied.
- **Goal Streaks—Daily Goals & Habits Tracker.** This app, available for the iPhone, iPod, and iPad, allows you to set goals and then track how long you can keep them going (i.e., create a "streak"). It allows you to set daily goals, but you can also set a goal of doing something several times a week (e.g., "Eat at home at least 4 nights a week") and track how long you can keep the streak going. It lends itself to any number of response inhibition goals.
- **StickK.com.** If you want to raise the stakes a little on your impulse control goal, check out the website *StickK.com*. Created by a Yale economist, Ian Ayres, the site is built around the notion of "commitment contracts," which is a variation on correspondence training, discussed in Step 7. There are four steps to the process, clearly

outlined on the StickK website: (1) Set a goal ("What do you want to achieve and what time frame will you give yourself to achieve it?"). (2) Set the stakes (This part is optional: "As an added incentive to succeed, do you want to lay money on the line? If so, how much? If you fail, where do you want that money to go?" People often choose to make a donation to a cause they strongly dislike). (3) Choose a referee ("Who do you want to designate to monitor your progress and confirm the truth of your reports to stickK?" This too can be optional, but finding a referee increases the likelihood that you're honest in your self-assessments). (4) Enlist supporters ("Who do you want to have cheering you on?"). It costs nothing to create a commitment contract. Check out the website to see the wide variety of goals people have set—it may give you some ideas!

Working Memory

There are a million to-do list and checklist apps out there. Find one that appeals to you.

- Our favorite is **Wunderlist.** It's a free app available for both iPhone and Android that allows you to create lists and access them across platforms. This can be particularly useful for household chores and repairs, shopping, and items needed for work, recreation, or exercise. You can also program reminders if needed.

- Another highly useful technological application is **Instapaper.** This program, which also works across platforms, is a way to store and manage all those interesting websites or articles you run into on the Internet. When you find something you want to save, you just save to Instapaper (it can be one of the items in your Bookmark Bar), and it automatically saves it in your Instapaper account. You can then organize everything you've saved in separate files. You can, for example, have files for personal information (e.g., exercise routines, recipes, and shopping). Each item has a hyperlink attached to it that gets you to the original website instantly and is listed by name as well as with a brief description to remind you what it is and why you saved it.

How about apps that help you find things you've misplaced?

- The **Find My iPhone** app can save you lots of time and grief. If you link technological equipment through Bluetooth, if you lose any one item (iPhone, iPad, or Apple laptop), you can track it down just by going to the Find My iPhone app on whichever device is available. You can instruct the app to play a sound on the missing device, and as long as your device is connected to the Internet, you will be able to locate it.

- Another piece of technology that falls into the find-lost-items category is **Tile** (*thetileapp.com*). Tiles are 1-inch-square devices that can be attached to a key ring or glued to a device (e.g., a TV remote) or just placed in a purse or suitcase. Each tile is labeled and programmed separately, and if the desired item goes missing, you can locate it using your smart phone. It will either show you on a map where the lost item is or make a sound so that if it's nearby you can locate it that way.

Emotional Control/Stress Tolerance

To be clear here, we consider emotional control and stress tolerance to be separate and distinct executive skills. As we have noted, however, apps and strategies are often relevant to more than one skill. An increasing number of apps are available to enhance emotional control and stress tolerance. We have focused here on relaxation strategies including meditation since they have a proven and in many cases evidenced-based track record. Breathe2Relax, Happify, and Headspace have been reviewed and recommended by the Anxiety and Depression Association of America (*https://adaa.org/finding-help/mobile-apps*#). Additional apps can be found on this website.

- One of our favorite apps for meditation is **Headspace,** which can be accessed either online (*headspace.com*) or through the App Store. As discussed earlier, this site features a former Buddhist monk named Andy Puddicombe, who leads daily guided meditation sessions. It is a subscription service, but the first 10 days are free, so the listener can decide whether it is worth purchasing a year's subscription. In the moment, meditation can be incredibly relaxing. It offers a brief respite from the busy, multitasking world we live in. If emotional control is a weak executive skill, the benefits of mindfulness meditation are particularly applicable. There is also evidence, however, that mindfulness can improve sustained attention, response inhibition, and flexibility.
- **Chillax** (*https://itunes.apple.com/us/app/chillax/id494538881?mt=8*). This is a free app that "uses a combination of soothing music, relaxing sounds, and binaural bests to ease you into a state of relaxation and calm." If you develop a coping strategy that involves taking a "time-out" to calm down or recover from a stressful experience, this might help.
- **Balanced** (*https://itunes.apple.com/us/app/balanced-goals-habits-motivation/id630 868758?mt=8*). This is a pretty straightforward app for setting goals and keeping track of personal improvement efforts. Many of the categories and choices relate to improving emotional control or personal well-being.
- **Breathe2Relax** (*https://itunes.apple.com/us/app/breathe2relax/id425720246?mt=8*). This app was developed by the National Center for Telehealth and Technology. Reading materials, a video demo, and progress charts are available and can be personalized by users. Breathing techniques are simple to develop with practice and have been validated for anxiety and stress reduction.
- **Happify** (*www.happify.com*). The objective of this app is to enhance positive emotions through the use of games and exercises supported by research in mindfulness meditation and positive psychology. Specific paths are suggested for the user from

the results of an initial questionnaire. Activities are geared to varied aims such as anxiety reduction, relationship building, improvements in fitness, and chronic-pain coping strategies. These activities include brief research findings or the scientific rationale for use. The app is initially free and includes paid upgrades.

Task Initiation

We referred to apps and smart phone use earlier, but we want to emphasize using technology both as an environmental support and as a vehicle for ensuring we practice the skill. Here are some options (of the hundreds available in the productivity section of your Apple or Google app store):

- **iSecretary.** This is an app for iPhone and iPad that allows you to record a voice memo and then have it play back at a designated time. It could remind you, for instance, to start your task initiation practice session at the designated time.

- **The Habit Factor.** This is an iPhone app that allows you to set goals related to building habits, remind yourself of those goals, and track your progress. You can select start and end dates (or keep it open ended), and you can designate which days you intend to practice the habit. There is a free version as well as one that costs a nominal amount.

- The alarm on your smart phone. This is the easiest device to use, and it comes with your phone. Just program your phone to remind you to start the task. You can set a recurring reminder or program it for a different time every day if you need to. One person we know uses the "snooze" function in a clever way. When the alarm goes off, if he can't get to it right then, he doesn't turn off the alarm; he hits snooze instead, which means every 10 minutes or so the alarm will go off again until he actually begins the task as intended. Better than a nagging spouse or parent, but the cues keep coming until you actually begin the task. (Colin continues to use these alarms on a daily basis.)

Sustained Attention

In addition to smart phone alarms and timers, here are some apps you may want to look at (selected from the hundreds available in the productivity section of your app store):

- **Pomodoro.** This is an iPhone or iPad app that can be used to implement the time management technique called "Pomodoro." We include it here because breaking tasks into segments is an effective strategy for sustaining attention. The technique (explained at *pomodorotechnique.com*) is built on breaking work down into 25-minute segments, followed by 5-minute breaks. When you've completed four time segments, called "pomodoros," you give yourself a longer break (e.g., 20 or 30 minutes). The term *pomodoro* is Italian for tomato, and if you visit the website, you can learn more about the technique, order the book that describes it in more detail, and purchase a timer that looks like a tomato!

- **iEarned That!** We could put this app under any of the executive skills, but we'll mention it here. It's intended for use with children and enables them to earn rewards in exchange for completing tasks. If you're reading this book, you're not a child, but if you have a sense of humor you might enjoy this app anyway. You take a picture of the reward you want to earn and turn the picture into a jigsaw puzzle with as few or as many pieces as you choose. Each time you complete a segment of a task (such as a practice session), you give yourself a puzzle piece. When the puzzle is complete, you earn the reward pictured on the puzzle.

Planning

There are more apps for planning for smart phones, tablets, and laptops than can easily be counted. Some are free, while others, especially those targeting a business clientele, can cost $100 or more. There are many geared to specific kinds of planning, such as wedding planning, meal planning, financial planning, travel planning (routes and checklists), and home decorating. If you think you might like to go the electronic route for planning, we recommend that you start by downloading one of the free apps (or the free versions of apps) to try them out before spending any money. Some are complicated, and many assume you have good planning skills to start with—these, for example, begin with identifying the sequence of steps that need to be followed. The advantage of an electronic app is that you can program alarms and reminders.

If, after trying a free version, you decide the app is the way to go, read the reviews for the app you're considering. Look at how much technical support the app provides you and whether reviewers describe the app using terms such as "intuitive" or "user-friendly." You may want to take a look at apps developed by Omnigroup (*omnigroup. com*). Of the ones we looked at, this one offers more detailed explanations and videos to help the purchaser understand how to use the various apps offered. Although Omnigroup has project management apps aimed at businesses that are fairly complicated, the **Omnifocus** app seems to be geared more to general use, applicable to both home and work projects.

As an alternative to **Omnifocus,** you may want to look at David Allen's materials. David Allen is a time efficiency expert who developed an approach called Getting Things Done (GTD). He has an enthusiastic following, and if you visit his website you can learn about training opportunities, podcasts, services, and products that explain and support his system. If you want a more objective appraisal of how well his system works, we recommend you go to Amazon and check the reader reviews for his book *Getting Things Done: The Art of Stress-Free Productivity*. There are almost 1,400 reader reviews, over half of which gave the book a 5-star rating. One 5-star reviewer wrote, "This book has changed my approach to my work life." But if you're skeptical that a book could do that, look at the more critical reviews. One wrote, "I never finished reading this book. I am a failure at getting things done."

What struck us as we checked out apps and looked at technology options is that there is no system out there that works perfectly for everybody. And keep in mind that most systems and apps were probably developed by people who were naturally good at planning and/or naturally good at navigating fairly complicated technology. If you do not fall into one or both of these categories, spend your money carefully.

Organization

- **HomeRoutines.** This app allows you to create routine checklists for daily and weekly household chores. The best part of the app, though, is that it builds in detailed cleaning lists, tied to different "Focus Zones." It also includes a built-in timer that you can set to 10 or 15 minutes that can be spent on "speed cleaning." Finally, it has built-in to-do lists for one-off jobs, but the whole app can be customized to fit your needs.

- **Cozi Family Organizer.** Available for iPhone and iPad, this is a color-coded family calendar that can be shared among family members that tracks schedules for the whole family all in one place. It also includes shopping lists and to-do lists that can be shared, allows one to set reminders to make sure people remember what's on the schedule, and will e-mail an agenda for the upcoming week to family members.

- **Inbox.** This is an e-mail management system that works on Google Chrome. It sorts your e-mails into categories such as Travel, Purchases, Promos, Social (i.e., social media such as Facebook), and gives you the option of dealing with the e-mail right away or choosing the "Snooze" function, which gets it off the e-mail list until you tell **Inbox** to bring it back. This last function ends up being very satisfying to people who feel compelled to clean out the e-mail folder every day but want to postpone responding to the e-mail until a later time.

Time Management

- **Pomodoro.** We described this technique/app in the Sustained Attention section, but it's worth mentioning again here. Breaking your work day into 25-minute segments with 5-minute breaks may help you learn to manage your time more effectively, especially if you combine it with practice estimating how much you can accomplish in each 25-minute segment. Check out the website *pomodorotechnique.com* for more information.

- **ATracker/ATracker PRO** is an iPhone or iPad app that enables you to track how you spend your time based on your own customizable categories. It's easy to set up, you can set alarms to prompt you to begin an activity at a certain time, and you can easily track how much time you spend on any activity by tapping the activity to start and stop it.

- **Rescue Time** is a desktop application that keeps track of how you spend your time across the workday. It records what websites you visit and tracks how long you spend on each at any given time. There's a free version as well as a paid subscription service that issues weekly reports with time breakdowns. It classifies websites as either productive or wasteful and lets you know how much time you spend on each one. You can also set goals and limit your access to wasteful sites according to your own rules.

Goal-Directed Persistence

As in the case with planning, there are a large number of apps devoted to goal achievement, some free and some quite expensive. If you think you want to go the app route for goals, we recommend that you start by downloading one of the free apps (or the free versions of apps) to try them out before spending any money. Some are complicated, and many assume you have good goal-setting skills to start with. The advantage of an app is that you can program alarms and reminders. If, after trying a free version, you decide an app is the way to go, read the reviews for any app you're considering. Look at how much technical support the app provides you and whether reviewers describe the app using terms such as "intuitive" or "user-friendly." The first three here were selected from the website *https://beebom.com/best-goal-setting-apps*. Given that planning is a key feature of goal attainment, these apps can also assist with planning.

- **The Habit Factor.** We mentioned this iPhone app under Task Initiation, but it fits well here also. This app allows you to set goals related to building habits, remind yourself of those goals, and track progress. You can select start and end dates (or keep it open ended), and you can designate which days you intend to practice the habit. There is a free version as well as one that costs a nominal amount.
- **Habitica.** For those who enjoy games, this free app for iPhone and Android lets you embed your goals into a role-playing game format. The app includes three types of tasks, Dailies, Habits, and To-Dos, and includes a rewards-and-punishments feature that can be a source of motivation for some people. Details can be found at *https://habitica.com*.
- **HabitHub** is described in reviews as a simpler goal app. It is not game based but has a graphic feature for easy tracking of progress and allows you to customize your own rewards. This app is free for Android devices, and at the time of this writing is coming for iPhone.
- **WOOP.** The term "WOOP" stands for wish, outcome, obstacle, plan. This app was developed by Gabriele Oettigen, a professor of psychology at New York University and the University of Hamburg (see Books section, p. 267). The app incorporates the research and clinical work of Oettigen and others at New York University. The app is unique in that it has been validated extensively in research and clinical settings for its effectiveness in helping people to achieve

their goals. It incorporates the techniques of implementation intentions with mental contrasting that we recommended in this book. The app is available as a free download for iPhone and Android. If you are interested in a goal achievement app, we highly recommend WOOP. See *http://woopmylife.org/app*.

Flexibility

Research suggests that meditation can increase flexibility (along with a number of other executive skills). We've described apps for meditation under Emotional Control.

- Here's a fun app for adjusting to unanticipated events. It's called **Make Dice**, and you can label the sides of a die with different tasks (chores or fun things to do) and then roll the dice to see what comes up first. This might also be a fun app for a family with kids as a way to divide up household chores among several family members. Each member can roll the die to see what chore he or she has to do that day.

- There's evidence to suggest that cognitive flexibility can be increased through playing real-time strategy video games. One of the biggest raps against brain training games is that if there are any benefits from playing them, they are most likely to show up on improved game performance and do not generalize to real-world applications. One recent study done with college students found that students who played the game "StarCraft" for 40 hours improved on other tests of cognitive flexibility. Admittedly, these tests were lab tests—such as the Stroop, which requires the subject to read as quickly as possible color words when the colors and the words don't match and the color the word is printed in has to be ignored to read the word correctly. Nonetheless, they are quite dissimilar from the video game that students were playing and are generally considered good measures of cognitive flexibility in that they require the test taker to rapidly switch between contexts. Unfortunately, most real-time strategy games are war games and may be more appealing to some individuals than others.

Metacognition

We are not aware of any specific apps that address metacognition. However, self-monitoring is a component of metacognition, and there are self-monitoring apps, although they tend to be devoted to student behaviors. Nonetheless, some of them may be adaptable to adult behaviors. In addition, if a parent or young adult has identified a different executive skill weakness, apps to improve that weakness will also have the benefit of increasing self-awareness of one's behavior, which is central to metacognition.

Index

Acceptance. *See also* Parental supports
  overview, 50, 53–57
  parental supports and, 52
  stepping aside and, 56–57
Accountability, 193
Acquisition of executive skills, 22–23. *See also* Development of executive skills; Executive skills
Action Plan for Achieving a Short-Term SMART Goal form, 171
Action steps
  Action Plan for Achieving a Short-Term SMART Goal form, 171
  challenges to achieving goals and, 179
  creating a plan to achieve goals and, 164–165, 166, 168
  SMART goals and, 158–161
  stuckness and, 223
Affirmation, 115
Alarm systems, 211, 212
Ambivalence, 44–45
"American Dream," 58–59
Anger, 236
Ansell-Casey Life Skills Assessment, 254
Anticipating challenges, 9. *See also* Challenges to achieving goals
Anxiety
  professional help and, 10
  psychological issues and, 236–238
  stalls and, 8
  when you aren't sure if a goal is a good fit, 132
Apartments, 259

Appointments, 257–258
Aptitudes
  goal attainment and, 16
  goodness of fit and goal setting and, 126
  identifying, 8–9
  readiness for change and, 59
Assessment, 26, 30–34
Assumptions, 13, 91
ATM use, 256–257
Attainable goals, 159, 161. *See also* Goals; SMART goals
Attention, sustained. *See* Sustained attention
Auto insurance, 260–261
Automobiles, 260–261

B

Banking services, 256–257
Benefits Provided by Parents to Young Adults checklist, 154, 155
Blame, 36, 115
Boundaries, 112–114, 219–220
Brain factors, 8, 23, 25

C

Career
  coaching and, 232–233
  goodness of fit and goal setting and, 121, 125, 126–129

Career *(cont.)*
  identifying or finding goals related to,
    106–109
  long-term goals and, 45–48
  Relationship-Based Executive Skills
    Questionnaire and, 106–109
Cars, 260–261
Cell phones, 263
Challenges to achieving goals. *See also* Goals
  environmental modifications and, 180–188
  overview, 177–180
  troubleshooting, 195–196
Change, 215–216, 228–230. *See also* Readiness
    for change
Change talk, 53–57
Choices
  challenges to achieving goals and, 178
  Getting to Know Myself Questionnaire
    (GTKMQ) and, 76–77
  task modification and, 186
  young adult's ownership of, 48–49
Coaching, 9–10, 230–235, 261–262
Cognitive techniques, 199
Collaboration
  adult children living with parents and, 64
  coaching and, 230–235
  goodness of fit and goal setting and, 134–135
  overview, 34–36, 39
  parental supports and, 51–52
  rather than coercion, 114–117
  time limits and, 118–119
  when you aren't sure if a goal is a good fit,
    131–132
College independence
  defining independence and, 42
  fading of the "American Dream" and, 58–59
  parental supports and, 52–53
College-related goals. *See also* Goals
  executive skills weaknesses and, 82
  Getting to Know Myself Questionnaire
    (GTKMQ) and, 80–81
  goal setting and, 127–131, 136–137
  Relationship-Based Executive Skills
    Questionnaire and, 109–110
  thinking through the challenges before
    planning, 137
Comfort with situation, 8
Communication
  about expectations and roles, 39
  conflicts and, 89–91

defining independence and, 39–42, 43
  Getting to Know Myself Questionnaire
    (GTKMQ) and, 76, 86–87
  identifying similarities and differences and,
    99–103
  managing differences in executive skills and,
    104–105
  rather than coercion, 114–117
  Relationship-Based Executive Skills
    Questionnaire and, 98–99
  when you aren't sure if a goal is a good fit,
    131–132
Community resources, 253–263
Confidence, lack of
  Getting to Know Myself Questionnaire
    (GTKMQ) and, 77
  learning from successes and, 243
  parental supports and, 53–57
  readiness for change and, 59, 60
  stalls and, 8
Correspondence training, 193. *See also*
    Education-related goals
Costs required to attain goals, 136–137
Credentials required to attain goals, 136–137
Credit and debit cards, 256–257
Criticism, 52

D

vvDaily living goals, 172–174
Deadlines. *See* Time urgency/deadlines
Debt issues, 256–257, 263
Decision making
  adult children living with parents and, 64
  seeking help from others and, 187–188
Delayed gratification
  goal-directed persistence and, 214
  response inhibition and, 199
Dental care, 257–258
Depression
  professional help and, 10
  psychological issues and, 236–238
  stalls and, 8
Development of executive skills, 22–25. *See also*
    Acquisition of executive skills; Executive
    skills
Discouragement, 53–57
Distractions, 195
Dream goals, 69–70. *See also* Goals

E

Eating habits, 236
Economic climate, 58–59
Education loans, 263
Education-related goals. *See also* College-related
    goals; Goals
  correspondence training and, 193
  executive skills weaknesses and, 82
  Getting to Know Myself Questionnaire
    (GTKMQ) and, 80–81
  goodness of fit and goal setting and, 127–131
  Relationship-Based Executive Skills
    Questionnaire and, 109–110
Effort, 196
Emotional control. *See also* Executive skills
  environmental modifications and, 182
  overview, 27
  Relationship-Based Executive Skills
    Questionnaire and, 93–94
  strategies to use to address weaknesses in,
    201–203
  technological resources to help with, 271
Emotional support, 50–51, 53–57. *See also*
    Parental supports
Employment
  fading of the "American Dream" and, 58–59
  finding a job, 258–259
  metacognition weaknesses and, 216–217
  SMART goals and, 172–174
"Empty-nest syndrome," 44
Encouragement, 50–51
Energy
  psychological issues and, 236
  troubleshooting and, 196
Environment. *See also* Environmental
    modifications
  anticipating trouble and, 9
  executive skill acquisition and, 22
Environmental modifications. *See also*
    Environment
  emotional control and, 201–203
  flexibility and, 215–216
  goal-directed persistence and, 212–214
  metacognition and, 216–218
  organization and, 209–211
  overview, 180–188, 198
  planning and, 207–209
  response inhibition and, 198–199
  stress tolerance and, 218–220

  sustained attention and, 205–207
  task initiation and, 204–205
  time management, 211–212
  working memory and, 200–201
Estimation of time, 212. *See also* Time
    management
Evaluating Success with Achieving SMART
    Goals form, 175
Executive skills. *See also* Acquisition of
    executive skills; Development of executive
    skills; Executive skills weaknesses;
    individual skills
  acquisition of, 22–23
  assessing in the young adult, 26, 30–34
  evaluating SMART goals and, 176
  Getting to Know Myself Questionnaire
    (GTKMQ) and, 70–71
  goodness of fit and goal setting and, 126
  identifying similarities and differences and,
    99–103
  identifying skills needed for independence
    and, 25–26, 27–29
  improving, 192–193
  overview, 16–17
  readiness for change and, 59
  Relationship-Based Executive Skills
    Questionnaire and, 92, 97–98
  seeking help from others and, 187
  troubleshooting and, 195–196
Executive Skills Definitions and Behaviors
    Checklist, 27–29
Executive Skills Questionnaire
  complete, 31–33
  learning from successes and, 248
  overview, 21, 30, 67
Executive skills weaknesses. *See also* Executive
    skills
  collaboration and, 34–36
  defining independence and, 40–41
  environmental modifications for, 180–188
  evaluating SMART goals and, 176
  goal selection and, 67–70, 82
  goal setting and, 147, 151
  identifying similarities and differences and,
    102–103
  learning from successes and, 240–250
  overview, 6–7, 15, 17–22, 220–221
  questions to ask yourselves regarding, 13
  seeking help from others and, 187
  stalls and, 7, 8

Executive skills weaknesses (cont.)
    strategies to use with specific weaknesses,
        182–184, 185–186, 197–221
    technological resources to help with, 269–276
    troubleshooting and, 195–196
Expectations
    communication regarding, 39
    defining independence and, 39–42, 43
    discouragement and lack of confidence and,
        53
    executive skills weaknesses and, 35–36
    goodness of fit and goal setting and, 127–129
    impetus for change, 230
    overview, 10, 90
    questions to ask yourselves regarding, 13
    stalls and, 7
Experience, 22
Expert opinion, 116
External factors, 58–59

F

Fantasy
    goal selection and, 69–70
    identifying or finding goals and, 110–112
    Relationship-Based Executive Skills
        Questionnaire and, 110–112
Financial management
    goal-directed persistence and, 212–214
    response inhibition and, 198–199
    tasks of independent living and, 256–257
    technological supports for, 212
    time management and, 212
Financial support. See also Parental supports
    overview, 51, 57–58
    stuckness and, 226, 227–228
    time limits and, 117–119
First–then schedules
    motivation and, 192
    troubleshooting and, 195
Flexibility. See also Executive skills
    environmental modifications and, 183
    goodness of fit and goal setting and, 127–129
    overview, 29, 215
    Relationship-Based Executive Skills
        Questionnaire and, 95–96
    strategies to use to address weaknesses in,
        215–216
    technological resources to help with, 276
Focus, 16, 51. See also Sustained attention

Forms/questionnaires/checklists
    Action Plan for Achieving a Short-Term
        SMART Goal form, 171
    Benefits Provided by Parents to Young
        Adults checklist, 155
    creating a plan to achieve goals and, 166, 168
    Evaluating Success with Achieving SMART
        Goals form, 175
    Executive Skills Definitions and Behaviors
        Checklist, 27–29
    Executive Skills Questionnaire, 31–33, 67
    Getting to Know Myself Questionnaire
        (GTKMQ), 70–71, 72–75, 76–77, 86–87
    How Do You Two Define Independence?
        checklist, 43
    Relationship-Based Executive Skills
        Questionnaire, 91–92, 93–96, 105–112
    SMART Goal-Setting Guide and
        Worksheet, 160, 162–163
    Summary Form: Helping Young Adults
        without a Goal Get Started, 143, 144–146,
        148–150
    Summary Form to Help You Assess
        Goodness of Fit, 122–124
Future, 45–48

G

Generating positive emotions, 191
Genetic factors, 22
Getting to Know Myself Questionnaire
    (GTKMQ)
    application examples of, 77–86, 87–88
    coaching and, 232
    communication and, 86–87
    complete, 72–75
    goodness of fit and goal setting and, 121, 125,
        128–129
    identifying a career path and, 108–109, 110,
        113
    lack of goals and, 140
    learning from successes and, 247
    overview, 70–71
    redoing when stuck, 223
    results from, 71, 76–77
    Summary Form to Help You Assess
        Goodness of Fit and, 122–124
Goal attainment. See also Goals
    challenges to, 177–180
    goal setting and, 147

learning from successes and, 240–250
writing down goals and, 161
Goal setting. *See also* Goals
  breaking down a goal and, 9, 156
  coaching and, 230–235
  examples of, 77–86
  goal selection and, 68–70
  goodness of fit and, 120–135
  overview, 9, 120, 147, 151
  parental supports and collaboration and,
    134–135
  SMART Goal-Setting Guide and Worksheet
    and, 160, 162–163
  Summary Form: Helping Young Adults
    without a Goal Get Started, 144–146,
    148–150
  thinking through the challenges before
    planning, 135–138
  time frames to complete goals and, 152–155
  when a goal does not seem like a good fit,
    121–125
  when a goal does seem like a good fit,
    125–131
  when you aren't sure if a goal is a good fit,
    131–135
  for young adults who don't have goals,
    138–147
Goal-directed persistence. *See also* Executive
    skills
  environmental modifications and, 184
  goal selection and, 68
  overview, 29, 212
  Relationship-Based Executive Skills
    Questionnaire and, 96
  strategies to use to address weaknesses in,
    212–214
  stuckness and, 224
  technological resources to help with,
    275–276
Goals. *See also* Challenges to achieving goals;
    Goal attainment; Goal setting; SMART
    goals
  adult children living with parents and, 63,
    64
  boundaries and, 112–114
  breaking down, 9, 156
  challenges to achieving, 177–180
  coaching and, 230–235
  creating a plan to achieve, 164–165, 166, 168
  defining independence and, 39–40
  development of executive skills and, 24

executive skills needed to accomplish, 16
executive skills weaknesses and, 34–35, 36
Getting to Know Myself Questionnaire
    (GTKMQ) and, 70–71, 76–77, 86
goodness of fit and, 67–70, 225–226
identifying or finding, 106–107
implementation of, 174–176
lack of, 138–147
lack of progress towards reaching, 222–230
learning from successes and, 240–250
overview, 7, 45–48, 222–223
parental coercion and, 62–63
parental supports and, 51–52
questions to ask yourselves regarding, 13
readiness for change and, 59
Relationship-Based Executive Skills
    Questionnaire and, 97, 105–112
short time horizon for, 117–119
stalls and, 7
time frames to complete, 117–119, 136–137,
    152–155
young adult's ownership of, 48–49
Goodness of fit
  goal selection and, 67–70
  goal setting and, 120–135
  stuckness and, 225–226, 227
  Summary Form to Help You Assess
    Goodness of Fit, 122–124
  when a goal does not seem like a good fit,
    121–125
  when a goal does seem like a good fit,
    125–131
  when you aren't sure if a goal is a good fit,
    131–135
Grocery shopping skills, 255–256
Guilt, 36

H

Health insurance, 257
"Helicopter" parents, 39–40
Help from others. *See also* Parental supports;
    Professional help
  learning from successes and, 244–245
  overview, 187–188, 189
  tasks of independent living and, 253–263
Hopelessness, 236
Housing, 259
How Do You Two Define Independence?
    checklist, 43, 50

I

Impetus for change, 228–230
Implementation intention, 194, 243
Incentives
    learning from successes and, 241
    motivation and, 188, 190–192
Independence. *See also* Independent living
        skills; Skills for independence
    adult children living with parents and,
        63–65
    boundaries and, 112–114
    communication about expectations and roles
        regarding, 39–42, 43
    overview, 222
    questions to ask yourselves regarding, 13
    time limits and, 117–119
    transitioning towards, 42, 44–48
    young adult's ownership of goals and, 48–49
Independence, skills for. *See* Skills for
        independence
Independent living skills. *See also*
        Independence; Skills for independence;
        Tasks of independent living
    defining independence and, 41–42
    executive skills needed for, 25–26, 27–29
    overview, 24–25
    resources to get help for, 253–263
    time frames to complete goals and, 154
Insurance, 257, 260–261
Interest
    coaching and, 232–233
    executive skills weaknesses and, 34–35
    Getting to Know Myself Questionnaire
        (GTKMQ) and, 70–71, 84, 85–86
    goals and, 16, 24, 45–46, 126
    goodness of fit and goal setting and, 126
    psychological issues and, 236
    stuckness and, 223–228
Irritability, 236

J

Job search strategies, 258–259. *See also*
        Employment

K

Knowledge, 126

L

Labeling, 115–116
Life skills. *See* Skills for independence
Limit setting
    impetus for change, 228–230
    stuckness and, 228
    time limits and, 117–119
Living skills. *See* Independent living skills
Living with parents. *See also* Parental supports
    conflicts and, 90–92
    recommendations regarding, 63–65
    time limits and, 117–119
Long-term goals. *See also* Goals; SMART
        goals
    coaching and, 233
    creating a plan to achieve, 166, 168
    learning from successes and, 243
    overview, 45–48, 157
    rewards and, 188, 190

M

Material support, 51, 57–58, 63–65. *See also*
        Parental supports
Measurable goals, 159, 161. *See also* Goals;
        SMART goals
Medical care, 257–258
Memory, working. *See* Working Memory
Mental contrasting
    learning from successes and, 243
    overview, 194
    troubleshooting and, 195
Mental health evaluations, 10. *See also*
        Psychological issues
Mental stimulation, 194, 243
Metacognition. *See also* Executive skills
    development of, 24
    environmental modifications and, 184
    overview, 29, 216, 239
    Relationship-Based Executive Skills
        Questionnaire and, 96
    strategies to use to address weaknesses in,
        216–218
    stuckness and, 224
    technological resources to help with, 276
Milestones, 157, 166, 168
Mismatches between skills and goals, 176
Mistakes, 52
Modeling of skills, 25

Money management. *See* Financial management
Moral support, 53–57. *See also* Parental supports
Motivation
adult children living with parents and, 63–65
assumptions regarding, 91
defining independence and, 41
executive skills weaknesses and, 34–35
Getting to Know Myself Questionnaire (GTKMQ) and, 77
goal setting and, 151
impetus for change, 228–230
lack of goals and, 138–147
long-term goals and, 45–48
overview, 36, 38, 59–63
parental supports and, 53–57
questions to ask yourselves regarding, 13
rewards as, 188, 190–192
stuckness and, 223–228
time frames to complete goals and, 152–153, 154
translating fantasy goals to attainable goals, 110–112
young adult's ownership of goals and, 48–49

N

Nervous system, 23
Neurobiology, 22

O

Offloading
organization and, 210–211
overview, 181
troubleshooting and, 195
working memory and, 201
Opinions, 98–99, 116
Optimism, 115–116
Organization. *See also* Executive skills
environmental modifications and, 183
overview, 28
Relationship-Based Executive Skills Questionnaire and, 95
strategies to use to address weaknesses in, 209–211
technological resources to help with, 274
working memory and, 201

P

Parent–adult child relationship
adult children living with parents and, 64–65
coaching and, 234
executive skills weaknesses and, 35–36
identifying similarities and differences and, 99–103
managing differences in executive skills and, 104–105
overview, 89–92
parental supports and, 51–52
Parental coercion
challenges to achieving goals and, 178–179
communication and collaboration in place of, 114–117
Getting to Know Myself Questionnaire (GTKMQ) and, 70
lack of goals and, 138–139
overview, 222–223
professional help and, 238
readiness for change and, 60–63
seeking help from others and, 187–188, 238
stuckness and, 226
Parental supports. *See also* Acceptance; Emotional support; Financial support; Material support; Moral support; Skill support
adult children living with parents and, 63–65
ambivalence regarding transitions towards independence and, 44–45
Benefits Provided by Parents to Young Adults checklist, 155
boundaries and, 112–114
collaboration and, 34–36, 51–52, 116–117
goodness of fit and goal setting and, 127, 134–135
identifying, 9
independent living skills and, 24–25
lack of goals and, 138–147
overview, 10, 49–59, 222–223
past successes, 52–53
providing the right level of supports, 58, 89–92
seeking help from others and, 187–188
stalls and, 8
stuckness and, 226, 227–228
tasks of independent living and, 253–263
thinking through the challenges before planning, 137
time frames to complete goals and, 117–119, 154

Parent-dictated goals. *See also* Goals
    executive skills weaknesses and, 35–36
    Getting to Know Myself Questionnaire
        (GTKMQ) and, 77
    overview, 60–63
    stalls and, 7
Parent's executive skills
    executive skills weaknesses and, 35–36
    identifying similarities and differences and,
        99–103
    managing differences in executive skills and,
        104–105
    overview, 90–92
    Relationship-Based Executive Skills
        Questionnaire and, 92, 97–98
Passion, 224–225. *See also* Interest
Patience, 88
Peer relations, 63–65
Performance feedback, 216–217
Periodic rewards, 191–192. *See also* Rewards
Persistence, 51
Physical environmental modifications, 182–184.
    See also Environmental modifications
Planning
    Action Plan for Achieving a Short-Term
        SMART Goal form, 171
    creating a plan to achieve goals, 164–165,
        166, 168
    overview, 16
Planning to achieve goals. *See also* Goals
    thinking through the challenges before
        planning, 135–138
    time frames to complete goals and, 152–155
Planning/prioritization. *See also* Executive skills
    environmental modifications and, 183
    overview, 28, 207
    parental supports and, 51
    Relationship-Based Executive Skills
        Questionnaire and, 94–95
    short-term horizon goals and, 119
    strategies to use to address weaknesses in,
        207–209
    stuckness and, 224
    technological resources to help with,
        273–274
Positive emotions, 191
Potential, 22
Predicting problems, 9. *See also* Challenges to
    achieving goals
Preferences, 8–9, 126–127
Preparation, 105

Privacy, 63–65
Problem-solving approaches
    challenges to achieving goals and, 178–179
    learning from successes and, 247
Procrastination. *See also* Task initiation
    impetus for change, 230
    strategies to use to address, 204–205
Professional help
    coaching and, 230–235
    overview, 9–10
    psychological issues and, 236–238
Prompts
    learning from successes and, 243
    troubleshooting and, 195
Psychological issues
    overview, 236–238
    professional help and, 10
    resources for, 263
    stalls and, 8
Public transportation, 260–261

R

Readiness for change. *See also* Change
    assumptions regarding, 91
    collaborative communication and, 116–117
    defining independence and, 41
    motivation and, 188
    overview, 36, 38, 59–63
    parental supports and, 113–114
Realistic goals, 159. *See also* Goals; SMART
    goals
Reflection, 116, 239–240
Regression, sense of, 63–65
Reinforcement, 50–51
Relationship-Based Executive Skills
        Questionnaire
    application examples of, 105–112
    communication regarding, 98–99
    complete, 93–96
    goal identification and, 105–112
    identifying similarities and differences and,
        99–103
    overview, 91–92
    seeking help from others and, 187
    using the information from, 97–98
Relationships between parents and adult
        children. *See* Parent–adult child
        relationship
Relaxation strategies, 196

Rescues, 8
Resolutions, 193–195
Resources
    books, 264–267
    magazines, periodicals, and newsletters, 267–268
    tasks of independent living and, 253–263
    technology, 269–276
    websites, 268–269
Response inhibition
    environmental modifications and, 182
    overview, 27, 198
    Relationship-Based Executive Skills Questionnaire and, 93
    strategies to use to address weaknesses in, 198–199
    technological resources to help with, 269–270
Rewards, 188, 190–192
Risk taking
    goodness of fit and goal setting and, 133
    parental supports and, 52
    psychological issues and, 236
Roles
    ambivalence regarding transitions towards independence and, 44–45
    collaboration and, 34–36
    communication regarding, 39
    defining independence and, 39–42, 43
    questions to ask yourselves regarding, 13
Roommates, 259

S

Sadness, 236
Seeking help from others. See Help from others
Self-awareness, 224
Self-determination, 224–225
Self-efficacy, 129, 191
Self-esteem, 129
Self-management, 235
Self-statements, 196
Sharing goals with others, 161
Shopping skills, 255–256
"Sink-or-swim" approach, 8
Skill building practices
    emotional control and, 201–203
    flexibility and, 215–216
    goal-directed persistence and, 212–214
    learning from successes and, 240–250

metacognition and, 216–218
organization and, 209–211
overview, 198
planning and, 207–209
response inhibition and, 198–199
stress tolerance and, 218–220
sustained attention and, 205–207
task initiation and, 204–205
time management, 211–212
working memory and, 200–201
Skill support. See also Parental supports
    adult children living with parents and, 63–64
    overview, 51, 57–58
Skills for independence. See also Independence; Independent living skills
    goodness of fit and goal setting and, 126
    overview, 8
    questions to ask yourselves regarding, 13
    specific weaknesses in, 9
    stuckness and, 226
Sleeping habits, 236
SMART goals. See also Goals
    action steps and, 158–161
    coaching and, 233–234
    creating a plan to achieve goals, 164–165, 166, 168
    daily living and work goals, 172–174
    deadlines for, 165–172
    Evaluating Success with Achieving SMART Goals form, 175
    examples of, 167–174
    learning from successes and, 243
    overview, 117, 151, 156–165, 160–161
    reviewing and clarifying, 174–176
    rewards and, 190
    stuckness and, 225–228
SMART Goal-Setting Guide and Worksheet, 160, 162–163
Social environmental modifications, 182–184. See also Environmental modifications
Soliciting help, 187–188, 189
Specific goals, 159. See also Goals; SMART goals
Spending behavior, 198–199
Stalls. See also Stuckness
    adult children living with parents and, 64
    anticipating and planning for, 177
    anxiety and, 132
    causes of, 7–8
Stepping aside, 56–57. See also Parental supports

Strengths
  identifying similarities and differences and, 101–102
  learning from successes and, 242
  managing differences in executive skills and, 104–105
Stress. *See also* Stress tolerance
  ambivalence regarding transitions towards independence and, 44–45
  psychological issues and, 236, 237
  troubleshooting and, 196
Stress tolerance. *See also* Executive skills; Stress
  environmental modifications and, 184
  overview, 29, 218
  Relationship-Based Executive Skills Questionnaire and, 96
  strategies to use to address weaknesses in, 218–220
  technological resources to help with, 271
Stuckness. *See also* Stalls
  coaching and, 230–235
  examples of, 225–228
  impetus for change, 228–230
  overview, 222–230
  psychological issues and, 236–238
Student loans, 263
Success, learning from, 10, 239–250
Summary Form: Helping Young Adults without a Goal Get Started, 143, 144–146, 148–150
Summary Form to Help You Assess Goodness of Fit, 122–124
Support from others, 187–188, 189
Supports from parents. *See* Parental supports
Sustained attention. *See also* Executive skills
  environmental modifications and, 183
  overview, 28, 205
  Relationship-Based Executive Skills Questionnaire and, 94
  short-term horizon goals and, 119
  strategies to use to address weaknesses in, 205–207
  technological resources to help with, 269–270, 272–273

T

Talent
  Getting to Know Myself Questionnaire (GTKMQ) and, 70–71
  goal attainment and, 16

Task demands, 176
Task initiation. *See also* Executive skills
  environmental modifications and, 183
  overview, 16, 27
  Relationship-Based Executive Skills Questionnaire and, 94
  short-term horizon goals and, 119
  strategies to use to address weaknesses in, 204–205
  task modification and, 185
  technological resources to help with, 272
Task modification, 185–186. *See also* Environmental modifications
Tasks of independent living, 8. *See also* Independent living skills
Technology
  coaching and, 235
  learning from successes and, 243
  offloading and, 181
  organization and, 210–211
  resources for, 269–276
  task modification and, 186
  time management and, 211
  troubleshooting and, 195
Temptation, 199
Time frames or limits required to attain goals
  goals and, 117–119
  impetus for change, 229–230
  negotiating deadlines and, 165–172
  overview, 136–137, 152–155
  short-term horizon goals and, 117–119
Time management. *See also* Executive skills
  environmental modifications and, 184
  overview, 28, 211
  parental supports and, 51
  Relationship-Based Executive Skills Questionnaire and, 95
  short-term horizon goals and, 119
  strategies to use to address weaknesses in, 211–212
  task modification and, 185
  technological resources to help with, 274–275
Time urgency/deadlines. *See also* Time management
  environmental modifications and, 184
  strategies to use to address weaknesses in, 211–212
Timely goals, 159. *See also* Goals; SMART goals
Tools, 25

Training, 129–131. *See also* Career; Education-related goals
Transportation, 260–261
Trust, 234

U

Undefined goals, 7. *See also* Goals

V

Variety, 186
Visualization, 190–191

W

Work goals. *See also* Employment
    finding a job, 258–259
    SMART goals and, 172–174
Working memory. *See also* Executive skills
    environmental modifications and, 182
    overview, 27, 200
    Relationship-Based Executive Skills
        Questionnaire and, 93
    strategies to use to address weaknesses in, 200–201
    sustained attention and, 206
    technological resources to help with, 270
Written plan, 63

About the Authors

Richard Guare, PhD, is Director of the Center for Learning and Attention Disorders in Portsmouth, New Hampshire.

Colin Guare, MS, is a registered behavior technician and writer who works with children and adolescents on the autism spectrum and is currently pursuing his board certification in applied behavior analysis (BCBA).

Peg Dawson, EdD, is a psychologist on the staff of Seacoast Mental Health Center in Portsmouth, New Hampshire. With decades of clinical experience, Peg Dawson and Richard Guare are coauthors of the bestselling *Smart but Scattered*, which focuses on younger children and preteens; *Smart but Scattered Teens* (with Colin Guare); and the adult-focused *Smart but Scattered Guide to Success*.